Herbal Healing Ground To Gut

"Unravelling the mysteries hidden in the ancient herbalism unknown to most people."

Willow Woman

Contents

Introduction

Herbal therapy has been practiced for thousands of years, and its existence predates today's pharmaceuticals. It is an essential part of complementary medicine, as it can help avoid and cure various illnesses. Nature's pharmacy is vast, brimming with herbs with potent healing properties. Everyone can use herbs to relieve pain and encourage recovery with the right advice and experience.

Plants have been used for food, medicine, lodging, clothes, dyes, firearms, musical instruments, and transportation since before recorded history. The knowledge and exploitation of plants have always been related to the cultural development of various countries and the rise and collapse of empires. Herbalism, or medicinal plants for the treatment, has long been practiced by all cultures. Our knowledge of herbalism has been passed on from generation to generation through word of mouth. Using local flora for food and medicine is the most natural thing globally, and recording this knowledge for posterity is the most natural thing in the world.

Both native peoples have a deep understanding of local herbs, and herbal knowledge is still used for primary healthcare in most parts of the world today. Shamans, wise women, bush physicians, herbal healers, and aboriginal medicine practitioners continue a thousands-year-old practice. Herbalism is the world's oldest, most tried, and validated method of medicine. The ancient Egyptians' Ebers Papyrus mentions 85 herbs, including mint, which are still used in similar ways today. About a thousand herbal treatments can be found in the Chinese herbal Pen, Tsao. Herbal recipes were written on clay tablets by Assyrian and Babylonian scribes. Herbs, cures, and therapy strategies listed by Hippocrates (477–360 B.C.E.) are still relevant today. There is a lot of practical and scientific wisdom that needs to be rediscovered. Herbal lore is a priceless treasure box all over the world.

The Leech Book of Bald, a combination of cures and ceremony, was written by the Saxons in the West. Yarrow, marigold, and hawthorn were among their nine sacred plants. They will also be highly regarded by a western herbal medicine practitioner. The invention of the printing press ushered in the glorious age of herbals. Culpeper wrote the London

Dispensary (1653) in English (it had previously been published in Latin) and later his Complete Herbal—a book in which every man (or woman) could learn how to treat themselves for less than three pennies, he boasted! Culpeper's herbal was a huge hit, and it is still available after more than 40 reprints.

For several years, botanical medicine was known as a type of alternative medicine. It was regarded as a valuable starting point for modern science, but it was dismissed as having little to give Western culture in terms of therapy. Pharmaceutical firms discovered the active therapeutic concepts in various plants, developed industrial analogs, and invented new medicines. However, they often ignored the most critical concepts of using natural sources for medicinal uses in the process. Herbalism, when done well, has a very different attitude to conventional medicine. Plants, or plant components, are used in a non-intrusive manner in a holistic system. Herbalists claim that a plant's constituents work together to enhance the body's internal healing mechanism.

Today, therapeutic programs that use plants as their primary source of treatment are seeing a worldwide revival. Traditional methods are being validated by modern science, prompting a general reappraisal. Tibetan, Chinese, Native American, Indian, and Western intellectual structures all explore their philosophical origins in a cross-cultural study that benefits everyone. Herbs are increasingly popular because they are perceived as a cleaner, cheaper, more sustainable, and have fewer side effects. This is not necessarily the case, though. An idiosyncratic reaction may be triggered by any substance. Herbs should be issued with caution and caution. We will improve our fitness, sense of identity, and enjoyment of living on the planet by following a few laws using common sense.

My mum, who used to be a herbalist healer, recently passed away, which is why I am writing this book. I was raised on seeing her practice herbal medicine throughout my childhood, and I want to follow in her footsteps. I have seen her make various medications from herbs and plants at home to treat multiple illnesses, such as homemade ice hot Neosporin, and so on. I saw her placing Amber bottles in the moonlight several times to pull out properties from the herbs and plants. I grew up hearing her tell stories about healers who were accused of being witches in the past when they used herbal treatments to cure different illnesses. Marijuana was once referred to as "the tree of life" by my mother, and I will explain why in later chapters. As she told me about her experience and expertise in this area, she learned the art and skills of preparing herbal medicines from a herbal healer academy and even read the herb Bible.

I will reveal the top-secret herbal curing plants and their effects on the human body, and how simple they are to cultivate. The majority of people today are unaware of the benefits of plants and herbs and how they are used for food. When they get ill, they look for prescription drugs. However, there are varieties of herbal remedies for various illnesses that can be used at home.

Plant sections in their fresh, natural state are used in specific herbal remedies. Some use store-bought extracts, and others require substances made in the warmth of your own home. I have effectively taken care of my own well-being and cure mild illnesses until they escalate and need medical attention by doing any testing, checking that a particular herb is correct and healthy for me, and taking all applicable safeguards. You can now do the same. Although medicinal herbs were once difficult to come by, they are now readily available in well-stocked pharmacies and on the shelves of big-box supermarkets. Whole spices, tinctures, teas, ointments, and other items are readily available in health food markets, making it easy to avoid pharmaceuticals.

It could confuse you to hear that a variety of traditional pharmaceuticals have their origins in herbal medicine. Willow bark is used to make aspirin, and opium poppies are used to make morphine. Quinine, a critical medication for malaria therapy, comes from the cinchona tree's bark, and digoxin, a powerful drug used in heart situations, comes from the beautiful yet toxic foxglove. Many other pharmaceuticals are derived from plants or made from molecules similar to those present in nature.

Despite this, synthetic medicines are preferred by conventional medicine due to their standardization, purity, and ease of use. Prescription pharmaceuticals, understandably, have a prized reputation. The aim of this book is not to minimize their significance. It is also worth remembering that in the United States, herbs are classified as dietary supplements and are treated as such when marketed commercially. As a result, you do not need a prescription to use an organic poultice, add a clear cream or oil, or take a tincture or tea anytime you decide to cure an ailment naturally, as you would for a synthetic medicine.

Though herbs are potent, they seldom have the long-term side effects that drugs do. They do not slow down the body's natural healing process; instead, they help us recover faster, particularly when combined with rest. Many herbs often strengthen the immune system, making it possible for the body to fight viruses and pathogens through its own defenses. It would take an enormous amount of time and money to catalog all of the world's medicinal plants, and even then, it would be almost difficult to cover all of the properties that each plant has to bring. Although there are many fantastic and comprehensive guides out there that outline hundreds of herbs, deciding which one to use can be difficult—especially when there are too many options.

This is a unique book. You can find a guide to using some of the world's most popular and potent medicinal herbs on these sites. They are both readily available online or at the nearest health food shop. It is also very likely that any of them would flourish within a short distance of your front door. Some of them may even be hidden in your spice drawer! This book would be helpful if you are new to herbal medicine or have already started to experience the healing potential of plants. The book's main section discusses specific diseases and remedies for each of them.

What Is Herbalism And How It All Started?

This chapter will include some background information on herbalism and its existence for centuries in almost every culture and area of the world. Herbs have played an important part in many cultures' medicinal practices since ancient times. This segment examines the main herbal systems that have existed throughout history in various parts of the world. Some of these structures can sound nonsensical to contemporary Westerners, but the alternative approach to health care that they embody may be just as real today as it was 5,000 years ago

Ancestries of Western Herbalism

For millennia, medieval Europe followed the teachings of Galen, a second-century physician who wrote widely about the body's four senses of humor – blood, phlegm, black bile, and yellow bile – and categorized herbs according to their essential qualities of hot, cold, dry, or moist. These ideas were later expanded by Arab physicians such as Avicenna in the seventh century, and Galenic theories still influence Unani medicine taught in the Muslim world and India today. Galen's definitions of herbs as "hot in the third degree" or "cold in the second degree" were also used in the eighteenth century.

Herbs in Ancient Civilizations

According to Egyptian papyri, many common herbs, such as garlic and juniper, have been used medicinally for about 4,000 years, dating back to 1700 BC. Indian hemp (marijuana) was used for eye conditions in the days of Ramesses III, just as it is now for glaucoma, and opium extracts were used to calm screaming girls. By Hippocrates' period (468–377 BC), European herbal tradition had already incorporated ideas from Assyria and India, with Eastern herbs like basil and ginger among the most highly regarded intricate principle of humor and vital body fluids had started to be developed. Hippocrates divided all foods and herbs into four categories: hot, cold, dry, and wet. Good health was achieved by maintaining a combination of these values and getting lots of exercises and fresh air. About 60 AD, Pedanius Dioscorides wrote the De Materia

Medica (Peri hulas iatrikes or About medicinal trees), which became the traditional textbook for the next 1,500 years. During Emperor Nero's reign, Dioscorides has been either Antony's and Cleopatra's physician or an army surgeon. Around 600 medicinal trees are covered with his herbal. Aromatics and "herbs with a sharp quality" were clustered together, as were appearances and parts used, such as stems, herbs, and "ground trees." Many of Dioscorides' actions are still practiced today: White horehound mixed with honey as an expectorant, parsley as a diuretic, fennel to stimulate milk flow, and parsley as a diuretic.

Roman Remedies

About 100 BC, Greek medical ideas entered Rome. They grew more mechanistic as time went by, portraying the body as a mechanism that needed to be constantly fixed rather than upholding the Hippocratic dictum that most ailments should heal themselves. With complicated and expensive herbal treatments, medicine became a lucrative industry. Claudius Galenus (131–199 AD), a court physician to Emperor Marcus Aurelius and a native of Pergamon in Asia Minor, was an outspoken opponent of the practice. Galen formalized the theories of humor and reworked much of the old Hippocratic ideas. His books quickly became traditional medical texts for Romans, but later Arab and medieval doctors and his teachings are still used in Unani medicine today.

Islamic Influences

With the fall of Rome in the fifth century, the emphasis on classical science moved East, with Constantinople and Persia being centers for the study of Galenical medicine. Galenism was enthusiastically accepted by Arabs in the Arab world, blended with folk traditions and surviving Egyptian learning. With the conquering Arab forces, this combination of medicinal ideas, practices, and customs was reintroduced into Europe. Avicenna's Kitab al-Qanun, or Canon of Medicine, was perhaps the most critical work of the period (Abdallah Ibn Sina, born at Bokhara in 910). This was founded on Galenical ideas, and by the twelfth century, it had been translated into Latin and reintroduced into Western medical schools as one of the most essential textbooks. Many herbs and spices from the East, such as nutmeg, garlic, saffron, and senna, were added to

Dioscorides and Galen's materia medica by the Arabs, who were excellent merchants.

The Greek Four-Element Model

The universe was divided into four elements by the ancient Greeks: earth, air, fire, and water. Seasons, the four essential qualities (hot, cold, dry, and damp), the four body fluids or humor, and the four temperaments were all linked to these elements. One humor was believed to predominate in nearly all people, influencing both appearance and the likelihood of health issues.

Blood, phlegm, black bile, and yellow bile were the four essential body fluids needed to be balanced to stay healthy. The temperaments – sanguine, phlegmatic, melancholic, or choleric – were linked to these. Since the melancholic humor was cold and dry, common ailments included constipation or intestinal upsets, which were treated with hot herbs to purge the melancholic humor and regain equilibrium. Senna and the Christmas rose (Helleborus niger), a harsh purgative, were both used to treat insanity and madness, all of which were attributed to a surplus of black bile and melancholy.

Cold and dampness dominated the phlegmatic personality, with typical ailments such as catarrh and chest problems. To maintain equilibrium and clear phlegm, warm and drying herbs like thyme and hyssop were used. On the other hand, the choleric temperament was thought to be "hot and dry" and was linked to poor temper and liver problems. To Clear Yellow Bile, Rhubarb Root, and other cool, moist plants like violets were used. The Galenical ideal was the Sanguine Person, Dominated by Heat and Damp: good-natured and entertaining, yet prone to overindulgence. Gout or diarrhea may be a concern, so herbs like burdock and figwort, which are cool and dry, can be used to stabilize the system.

A Science of Life

Ayurveda is derived from two Indian words: Ayur, life, and Veda, which means wisdom. As a result, Ayurvedic medicine is often referred to as "knowledge of how to live," stressing that good health is a personal obligation. In Ayurvedic medicine, the disease is seen as an imbalance, and herbs and dietary restrictions are used to maintain order. The first Ayurvedic texts date from about 2500 BC, with subsequent settlers introducing new medicinal traditions: the Persians in 500 BC; the Moghuls in the fourteenth century, who brought Galen and Avicenna's medicine (known as Unani medicine from ionic meaning Greek); and the British, who closed down the Ayurvedic schools in 1833 but fortunately did not obliterate the ancient learning entirely. Tibetan medicine has many similarities with Ayurveda, but it is much more complex, with 15 comedy subdivisions and a heavy focus on the impact of previous lives – karma – on current health.

Ayurvedic Principles

Like ancient Greek and traditional Chinese medicine, the Ayurvedic paradigm connects the microcosm of the organism with the universe. The three primal forces: prana – the breath of life; and – the spirit of light or fire; and soma – a representation of unity, cohesiveness, and compassion – are at the heart of the structure. All matter is made up of five elements: earth, water, fire, air, and ether (a nebulous nothingness that fills all space and is known to the ancient Greeks). The digestive fire (Agni) converts the five fundamental elements into three humors, which affect human wellbeing and disposition and are often referred to as waste products of digestion.

There would be no humoral imbalance if digestion were flawless, but imbalance and ill health can result since it isn't. Vata (wind) is created by combining air and ether, pitta (fire or bile) is created by combining earth and water, and Kapha is created by combining earth and water (phlegm). The prevailing humor is often thought to influence an individual's disposition: a Vata–style resembles Galen's melancholic personality, pitta–type corresponds to the choleric type, and a Kapha–resembles the phlegmatic type. Food, drink, sensual pleasure, light, fresh air, and spiritual practices are all used to "feed" the intestinal fire and produce the proper balance of humor.

Catarrh, edema, or water retention, for example, are handled with wet, light, and dry diets, fasting, and avoiding cold beverages, which improve Kapha. Pungent spices like cayenne, pippali, or cinnamon; bitters like aloe or turmeric; pungent tonics like saffron; and calming, mind-clearing herbs like Gotu kola, guggul, or myrrh are all herbal treatments for drying excess water or phlegm. Taste is essential in Ayurvedic theory: pungent, bitter, and astringent tastes may help to minimize Kapha, so sweet, salty, and sour flavors should be avoided in the diet. Massage with warm medicinal oils like eucalyptus; pungent smoking incense like frankincense; and urging the sufferer to wear vivid, hot reds and yellows instead of cool blue or white are all possible treatments.

Tibetan Herbalism

Tibetan medicine was mainly under the influence of the lamas and closely related to religion until the Chinese invasion in 1959. With the help of "illustrated trees of medicine," medical students memorized intricate "tantras" that clarified the origin and evolution of the disease. Each leaf represented a cause of disease, type of humor, effect, or result (such as the patient's age, his or her karma, the season of the disease, and so on). To "energize" the remedy and improve its potency, doctors used yoga and mantras. Herb harvesting was often deliberately timed to take advantage of any favorable astrological factors.

Chinese Herbal Medicine

Traditional Chinese medicine is a centuries-old healing system that dates back to about the year 2000 BC. Practitioners also study and practice the texts created at that time, and although much has been applied to the core theory, very little has been taken away. In Chinese medicine, the disease is seen as a symptom of general discord, so the traditional Chinese practitioner's job is to often restore peace and order. Herbs are at the heart of the procedure and are supplemented with various treatments, including acupuncture and professional massage. Chinese herbal practices have become more well-known over time, and many trained practitioners now use them.

Ancient Chinese Medicine

Chinese herbalism's beginnings are veiled in legend. Legendary figures include Shen Nong, the "divine cultivator," who named several medicinal plants. Shen Nong is known to have "tasted the flavor of hundreds of herbs and drank the water from many springs and wells so that people could know which were sweet and which were bitter." He has also explored tea drinking when several tea leaves dropped into a bowl of boiling water nearby. Shen Nong is an effective Chinese herbal (Shen Nong Ben Cao Jing), dating back to about 200 BC.

The "Yellow Emperor," who lived about 2500 BC, is considered the founder of Chinese medical theory. The Huang Ti Nei Ching Su Wên, or Yellow Emperor's Canon of Internal Medicine, is a classic text that bears his name and is usually dated to about 1000 BC. It may be a remnant of an earlier oral culture. Medicine, like medicine in the West, was inextricably linked to philosophy and theology at the time, and the Nei Ching is a significant Taoist text full of divine knowledge. In the past, China had a diverse range of medicinal philosophies and procedures, including a mixture of itinerant doctors, village herbalists, and native shamans. Taoist philosopher-doctors wrote classic medical texts that may have been the aristocracy's first preference in illness.

Modern Chinese Medicine

Western mission hospitals had started to represent a proper solution to conservative practices by the nineteenth century. Chinese medicine survived, but it was not until the 1960s that Mao Tse Tung founded five colleges of traditional Chinese medicine that it became a national medical system. Popular Korean, Vietnamese, and Japanese doctors also practice older ethnic healing methods, as do remaining Chinese medical families, many of whom have emigrated to Hong Kong, Singapore, or San Francisco.

The Principles of Chinese Medicine

Like early Greek philosophy, the Chinese culture was founded on a five-element principle, rather than the Greek four, which was used to describe any relationship between people and their surroundings. These elements – wood, fire, earth, metal, and water – are seen to be connected and linked to the seasonal cycle, with wood promoting fire, fire resolving to earth, earth yielding metal, metal creating water (seen as condensation on a cold metal surface), and water giving birth to wood by encouraging the growth of vegetation. None has been taken from ancient scriptures of traditional Chinese medicine, but a lot has been added. Each factor is linked to various things, including feelings and body parts, human sounds, seasons, colors, and tastes, all of which are based on basic logic. For instance, wood is associated with spring, germination, and the color green; fire is associated with summer, sun, and the color red; and water is associated with kidneys, winter, and the color black. The elements must balance good health to prevail; if one element becomes too dominant, the disease will result.

Chinese practitioners sometimes search for the source of illness in a related element: for example, liver weakness (wood) may be caused by kidney deficiencies (water). Over-exuberant wood (liver) failing to be managed by deficient metal could create a poor stomach (earth) (lungs).

Prescribing Herbs

The Chinese typically recommend herbs in traditional formulas (there are thousands in everyday use), which can be tweaked somewhat based on the patient's particular case. The recipe may contain as little as two herbs or as many as twenty, and the relationship between them is just as important as their individual properties. The product is often a potent concoction that can have drastic medicinal effects but defies basic scientific understanding.

Herbs are often administered as tablets, powders, or decoctions known as "tang" or "soup," which patients prepare at home for an hour or so in a special earthenware crock held for the purpose. The herbs are often cooked with rice to make a cereal-like therapeutic meal. A plant's characteristics in traditional Chinese herbals often include flavor, dominant temperature, and a general indicator of the organ and channels it affects. These are usually clearly linked, e.g., Chinese goldthread (huang lian, Coptis Chinensis) is a bitter herb. It is cold and has a solid connection to the nucleus, all of which are features that can be traced back to the five-element form. It may be used to treat disorders like insomnia, palpitations, and hot flushes, which are all symptoms of too much heat in the heart, according to traditional Chinese medicine.

Many nutritious herbs, such as rice or oats, and major tonics, such as ginseng, are sweet and healthy for the stomach and spleen. At the same time, Bai Shao Yao (white peony, Paeonia lactiflora) is sour and commonly used for liver problems – both of which are aspects of the ingredient wood – while many nutritious herbs, such as rice or oats, and major tonics, such as gins In the Chinese model, the five elements are intertwined, with fire giving birth to earth, which gives birth to metal, and so on.

Out of the Dark Ages

The resulting "dark ages" did not fully submerge European herbal rites after the fall of Rome. The "barbarians" introduced their own herbal healing rituals to add to the Roman practices that remained. With the expansion of Christianity, there was a significant exchange of new drugs and tried and tested remedies. The Church was instrumental in planting physic gardens and adding fresh herbs during the medieval period. Classical wisdom extended from the cloister to supplement folk medicine and domestic herbal medicines handed down over the centuries with the invention of the printing press.

Expansion of Herbalism in Europe

The Anglo-Saxon Leech Book of Bald, Europe's oldest surviving herbal written in the vernacular, dates from the first half of the tenth century and contains remedies sent by the Patriarch of Jerusalem to King Alfred. A wide range of ailments caused by "flying venom" and "elf-shot," which were words used to describe a wide range of unexpected or wasting illnesses, are defined in detail. Wood betony, vervain, mugwort, plantain, and yarrow were among the most prevalent herbs in Saxon times, used in various internal remedies but most commonly worn as amulets to ward off the evil eye.

While medical schools sprang up all over Europe – the most notable of which was established in the early tenth century in Salerno and taught the Hippocratic ideals of a healthy diet, exercise, and fresh air – healing and herbalism mainly remained in possession of the Church, with all monasteries cultivating medicinal herbs and ministering to the sick as part of their Christian responsibilities. Healing was as much a matter of prayer as it was of medicine, and early herbalists would often mix divine incantations with infusions, concluding that the patient would be healed with "God's help.".

Health Care Evolves

When the study progressed away from the cloister, the healing skills and practices formerly taught at the Salerno school were eventually reintroduced. Paracelsus (born Philippus Theophrastus Bombastus von Hohenheim near Zürich in 1493) was changing European attitudes toward health care by the 1530s. He focused on lecturing in German rather than Latin because he was both an alchemist and a physician. Many apothecaries and doctors, he thought, were shady characters out to fleece the public. He encouraged a return to more specific drugs influenced by the Doctrine of Signatures, condemning the complicated and frequently dangerous purgatives and emetics they recommended.

Physicians such as William Turner adopted Paracelsus, writing in English so that "apothecaries and old wives that gather herbs" would know the plants physicians meant by their Latin prescriptions and would not place "many a good man jeopardy of his life" due to ignorance. Nicholas Culpeper (1616–1654) later took a similar stance, provoking the wrath of the College of Physicians by translating their Pharmacopoeia into English so that ordinary citizens could buy drugs in hedgerows instead of paying exorbitant apothecary bills.

Herbal Warfare

Throughout the seventeenth and eighteenth centuries, wars fought between herb wives, apothecaries, and physicians, as medicine became more firmly under the jurisdiction of academic physicians with their university training. At the same time, dispensing was strictly controlled by the apothecaries. The emphasis was on expensive and complex nostrums containing mercury and antimony and costly and difficult nostrums containing mercury and antimony.

Numerous new herbs were being introduced from the East Indies and North 'America by the time the great herbals of Gerard (1597), Parkinson (1640), and Culpeper (1653) were published. Plants like nasturtium (Tropaeolum majus), nutmeg, and yucca started to show up in herbals, often with creative applications and arguments for medicinal properties. Tea is a classic example, once hailed as a panacea in the seventeenth century but now dismissed by many as nothing more than a trendy beverage.

North American Traditions

The first European settlers in North America brought familiar medicinal plants from home, such as heartsease and plantain, known as "white man's foot," because it grew everywhere the settlers went. They have picked up on several Native American healing practices, learning about new plants like boneset, echinacea, goldenseal, and pleurisy root (Asclepias tuberosa). Several American tribes also made extensive use of sauna-like sweat houses, and Samuel Thomson and his disciples adopted the concept of fire as a curing tool. The Physiomedical and Eclectic schools arose from this blending of cultures, which were later introduced into Europe and have had a lasting impact on herbal practices in the United Kingdom.

Ritual Herbalism

Herbalism in Native America was shamanistic, focusing on the practices of the medicine man, or shaman. The shaman will reach a trance-like state by playing drums and rattles and smoking tobacco or peyote mixtures, allowing him to spirit-travel and seek out the dying person's soul to save and restore it. Shamans in South America still use grape extracts – known as yage in Colombia and ayahuasca in Peru and Ecuador – in the same way. Siberian shamans used to navigate by ingesting fly agaric toadstool, whereas European witches used poisonous nightshade, henbane, thorn apple, or mandrake to do so.

The medicine wheel was also used in Native American rituals, and animal totems were assigned to the four cardinal directions. They compared it to various personality forms, supernatural forces, illnesses, and herbal remedies. The coyote, for example, was traditionally associated with the details of prosperity and love in the South. In contrast, the eagle was associated with the powers of intelligence and enlightenment in the East. The medicine man will fly in these symbolic ways in his spirit journeys, searching for the dying person's soul. Sweat houses were also typical among many Indian tribes, who created a sauna-like atmosphere where sick people were forced to sweat to rid their bodies of toxins or bacteria.

From Plants to Pills

Orthodox herbalism has generally favored "whole" plants and used blends of herbs to alter results, even though extracts, such as essential oils, have been prepared from different plants for decades. The movement to extract and classify individual active ingredients, then use them as single drugs, started in the eighteenth century, and there are now tens of thousands of them. These compounds have properties that are very distinct from those of the herb. These experimental medicines were initially only available as plant extracts, but after the chemical properties of certain sections were discovered, the drugs could now be synthesized. Scientific medicine has lost the art of mixing herbs to alter toxicity and use whole plants, which have chemical additives that can reduce the risk of side effects and transition from wild plants to clinical tablets. Medicine has lost the art of mixing herbs to alter toxicity in the shift from wild plants to clinical tablets.

Herbs in Modern Medicine

Morphine, discovered in 1803 by Friedrich Wilhelm Serturner in Germany, was one of the first synthetic medicines to be isolated from plant material. From raw opium poppy, he removed white crystals. White crystals were quickly developed from crude opium poppy using similar techniques. Aconitine from monkshood, emetine from ipecacuanha, atropine from deadly nightshade, and quinine from Peruvian bark were created using similar techniques. These compounds are classified as alkaloids and highly potent, but before scientists could synthesize them, they could only be derived from raw plants.

Salicin, which had been known as one of the active ingredients in willow bark, was synthesized for the first time in 1852. In 1899, the pharmacy manufacturer Bayer introduced acetylsalicylic acid as aspirin, which was changed to be a less gastric irritant. Bean extracts are also widely available in pharmacies. Various ephedrine preparations are derived from ma huang (Ephedra sinica), both prescription and over-the-counter, primarily used to treat coughs, catarrh, hay fever, and asthma. Pilocarpine, derived from jaborandi, is used to treat glaucoma; vincristine, derived from the Madagascar periwinkle, is used to treat leukemia; and strophanthin, derived from Strophanthus kombé, used to tip poison arrows in tropical Africa, is used to treat severe heart disorders. Morphine was one of the first synthetic medicines isolated from plant products, extracted from the opium poppy.

Chemicals extracted from plants can be highly potent, causing side effects previously unexplained until the entire plant was used. For example, Indian snakeroot, Rauwolfia serpentina, has been used in Ayurvedic medicine for centuries to treat snakebites, nausea, headaches, fevers, and abdominal pains. If Mahatma Gandhi was overstimulated, he was said to drink snakeroot tea at night. It was valued as a potent tranquilizer in the West, and it was used for elevated blood pressure and schizophrenia, and insanity.

CIBA isolated the alkaloid reserpine from snakeroot in 1947 and started selling Serpasil as a hypertension treatment. On the other hand,

Reserpine has unfavorable side effects such as extreme depression and irregular heartbeat slowing. By the 1960s, the herb had been reduced to the level of a prescription-only medicine in the United Kingdom, essentially excluding herbalists from using it. Rauwolfia serpentina, on the other hand, is still commonly used in other areas of Europe and Asia, where it is regarded as a calming tranquilizer.

Medicinal Meals

Plant classification as spices, berries, fruits, and "weeds" is a relatively new concept. Cabbage, carrots, and cucumbers were all considered "kitchen herbs" in the seventeenth century, much like marigolds and marjoram. We also neglect that the active constituents of "herbs," such as alkaloids and saponins, are not limited to the plants we mark as such: fruits and vegetables may be therapeutic or harmful in abundance. Foods were categorized in the past by temperature or flavor and were matched to the body's needs to ensure equilibrium. Fresh foods, according to Hippocrates, "give more strength" because they are more alive, whereas

Tibetan medicine considers frozen foods to be cooler and heavier than their fresh counterparts.

Care and Cultivation

Since this book focuses on treatments and use, you will mostly find information on what ingredients you will need and where to get them. Here are some tips on cultivating, preserving, and extracting healing herbs for those of you with green thumbs.

Plant a Healthy Landscape

Many medicinal plants will draw pollinators and bring lovely colors to your home's landscape in addition to treating mild illnesses in your family. Focus on seasonal plants to will the number of planting tasks you have to do each year. Echinacea, bee balm, catnip, and lavender are all outstanding perennials to remember. Include any feverfew in your annual herb garden if you suffer from migraines.

Prepare Garden Beds

Prepare a growing space for your medicinal plants before you bring them home to ensure they remain well. Follow the planting directions to the letter, and keep an eye on them for the first week after transplanting since they may need extra water or shade before they settle in.

Save the Resources

Wildcrafting is a method in which uncultivated herbs, seeds, and even fungi are harvested from the wild, then replanted at home for new harvests. American ginseng and goldenseal are two examples of valuable herbs historically gathered from their natural environment in practice called wildcrafting. If you love using a particular herb but do not want to pay for it, read about its requirements and try cultivating it in your backyard. You can find seeds and rootstock online.

Plan Ahead

Learn as much as you can about the plants you want to pick from nature and go out of your way to find them before harvest time so you can keep an eye on them and harvest them at the optimal time. Before removing even a single plant, double-check that wildcrafting is permitted in the area where you want to grow your herbs and secure any required permits.

Get Educated

The dandelion is one of many medicinal herbs that are called weeds. Keep your lawn native and encourage plants like mullein, low-growing plantain, chickweed, and dandelion to mingle with your grass to easily wildcraft at home. Allow them to grow for a while, then harvest what you need and mow as normal. Without any commitment on your behalf, these hardy herbs will return year after year. Gather plants only in places where no herbicide or pesticide has been used to protect yourself.

The Science behind the Remedies

Many herbs and botanicals are used to make sure common medicines, as we have discovered. We will get into this further when we look at the treatments, so here's a quick rundown on what happens when you use herbal remedies.

Gastrointestinal Health and Good Liver Function

Herbal treatments also work best with minor stomach issues like indigestion and nausea. Often what you need is a cup of peppermint or chamomile tea to make you feel better. Overworked livers prosper as well, as many herbs provide protection and can also aid in the recovery of normal function after an accident or disease. A well-known example of a herb that will help keep the liver stable is milk thistle.

Immune Function, Infection, and Inflammation

Many botanical medicines boost the immune system, while others aid in infection prevention and inflammation reduction. Echinacea is an immune-stimulant herb that can avoid infection, while ginseng is a botanical that will help you stay well by boosting the immune system. Four of the best botanicals for suppressing inflammation are St. John's wort, ginger, and ginkgo Biloba.

Musculoskeletal Discomfort

Internal and external herbal remedies should be used to treat minor sprains, sore muscles, and swollen joints. Externally, herbs like calendula, witch hazel, and capsicum offer medicinal comfort; internally, botanicals with high levels of antioxidants help connective tissue protection.

Psychological, Neurological, and Behavioral Health

If you look at a commercial about a prescription drug that aims to promote mental health, you will find that most of them come with alerts about possible side effects. Herbal treatments like ginkgo Biloba and valerian will help restore equilibrium without creating any complications of their own.

Reproductive Health

When you know which herbs to use, premenstrual syndrome (PMS), menopause complications, and maternity side effects are also easier to treat. Morning vomiting can be relieved with ginger, and black cohosh can assist with PMS and menopause symptoms. Ginseng, ginkgo Biloba, and saw palmetto are only a few herbs that can help with male reproductive health.

Respiratory Health

Over-the-counter drugs are often used to treat sore throats, coughs, and colds, but they have unpleasant side effects. These irritations and stuffy sinuses, and mild respiratory infections also react well to herbal medicines. Echinacea is used to cure colds and flu, and thyme and hyssop can help alleviate bronchial spasms so you can sleep.

Herbal Remedies and Home Recipes for Various Ailments

Useful Herbal Remedies

Herbs are the only treatment for all forms of health conditions in many parts of the world. Though licensed herbalists in the West can use herbs to treat serious health issues, there is also a wide variety of gentler remedies that can be used at home to treat common maladies. This section contains preparation guidelines as well as an ailment-by-ailment map. Herbs that can be easily used at home as an alternative to over-the-counter medications are the priority. Where applicable, other widely prescribed herbs are included.

Harvesting & Drying Herbs

The constituent chemicals and, as a result, the medicinal properties of herbs can be significantly influenced by when and where they are harvested. In the past, elaborate rituals were practiced to ensure that plants were harvested while they were their most potent: at a certain moon period when the Dog Star could be seen or certain zodiac signs. These practices are also evident in Tibetan medicine, where herbs are often harvested at astrologically significant times for the patient. The most crucial factor for most herb gatherers is to gather the herbs on a dry day when the plant is at its height of growth, and the abundance of active ingredients is at its maximum.

Herbs should be dried as soon as possible and away from direct sunlight to conserve the aromatic components and avoid deterioration of other compounds. Good air circulation is also needed, so tie the flowers in small bunches and ensure good air circulation. It could be practical to use an airing cupboard with the door left open, a spare room, or a dry garden shed with a low-powered fan running. Avoid drying herbs in garages because diesel fumes can contaminate them. Herbs can be thoroughly dried in a few days; the longer they take to dry, they will more likely discolor and lose their taste. The ideal drying room temperature is between 20–32°C/70–90°F, with no temperature above 38°C/100°F.

When the herbs are dehydrated, store them in clean, dry, dark glass or pottery jars with an airtight lid and keep them out of direct sunlight. The herbs can mold if they are handled while they are still slightly moist. Dry spices should be labeled with the type, source, and date. If properly dried and preserved, most can last 12–18 months without significant degradation.

Flowers

When the flowers are completely open and the morning dew has evaporated harvest. Handle with caution because they are easily harmed. Large flowers should have their stems chopped off. Small flowers (like lavender) may be dried on their branches, but if the stalk is fleshy, like mullein's, the flowers must be cut and dried separately. Remove any visible soil, grit, or insects from the flower heads and lay them out on newspaper or trays to dry in the airing cupboard or a warm sunny spare bedroom. Store flower petals in dark glass or pottery containers or in cabinets until dried, as the sunlight quickly deteriorates flower petals. Small flowers may be kept whole, but marigold petals should be removed from flower heads after drying and the center of the flower discarded. Lavender flowers should be dried in a paper bag or over a tray like seeds.

Aerial Parts and Leaves

Large leaves (like burdock) should be collected and dried separately, but smaller plates (like a lemon balm). Generally, deciduous herbs' leaves can be harvested only before flowering, while evergreen herbs like rosemary can be harvested all year. Coltsfoot leaves emerge after the flowers have bloomed and should be collected at that time. If you are going to use all of the aerial parts, the best time to order is when the plant is in the middle of flowering, so you get a combination of leaves, stems, fruits, and seed heads.

Hang upside down in small bunches of around 6–10 stems, depending on height. The herb is ready when the leaves are brittle but not so dry that they turn to powder when touched. Remove any significant bits of the stem from the stem and rub them onto paper or into a basin. If all of a plant's aerial components are being used, collapse everything together. Fill an airtight, opaque jar halfway with dried herbs.

Seeds

Harvest when mature, or when two-thirds of the seeds on a large seed head, such as fennel, are ripe, and before too many have been scattered by birds or the wind. Large seed heads with around 15–25 cm of the stem should be gathered and dried in small bunches.

Hang the bunch over paper or wrap it in a paper bag that is loosely bound to the bunch. When the seeds are mature, they can fall off and be collected in the bag over the next few weeks. Keep in a dark, airtight jar.

Root

Roots are typically harvested in the autumn when the plant's aerial parts are no longer in use. Roots are usually collected in the fall when the plant's aerial parts have died down and the earth has hardened sufficiently to make digging impossible. Dandelion stems, on the other hand, can be harvested in the spring. To clear dust and debris from the roots, vigorously wash them. Large roots can be sliced into small pieces when still young, as cutting them when dry can be difficult.

Spread the parts on trays and dry in a very cold oven for 2–3 hours (repeat this step two to three times for larger roots, but search frequently to prevent carbonizing the pieces), then move to an airing cupboard or a dark sunny space to finish drying undisturbed. Roots should be kept dry and airtight-free from direct sunshine. Some retain moisture from the air after drying and should be discarded if they become soft.

Saps and Resin

These can be obtained from trees by cutting a deep incision in the bark during the autumn sap flow and storing the sap in a cup attached to the flower. A large bucket can be required; for example, large volumes of birch sap may be gathered overnight at some times of the year. Since certain saps are corrosive, gloves should be worn. Squeezing the leaf stems of plants like lettuce and greater celandine over a bowl may be used to gather sap, but small quantities can normally be squeezed directly from the plant if desired. Splitting open an aloe leaf and pouring the gel it holds into a cup with a palette knife or spatula is how you get aloe sap.

Fruit

Berries and other fruits should be picked while they are only ripe until they get too soft or pulpy to dry. Spread out on trays to dry in an airing cupboard or a warm place. Fleshy fruits should be turned daily to ensure even drying, and those that show signs of mold should be discarded.

Bark

To avoid causing harm to the fruit, the bark should be harvested in the autumn while the sap is falling. If you wish to sacrifice the plant to herbal medicine, never cut any of the bark – or a band of bark covering a tree. To kill moss or insects, dust, or clean the bark, please do not soak it in water. Break into manageable parts (2–5 cm sq.) and place on trays to dry in an airing cupboard or a dark, dry, airy space.

Bulbs and Corms

After the aerial parts have died down, harvests are made. Harvest garlic corms as soon as the aerial portions of the plant have settled down.

Garlic corms should be collected as soon as possible after the leaves have wilted, as they begin to migrate downward and can be difficult to spot.

Supplementary Herbal Remedies

Massage Oils

Essential oils should be filtered before being used for massage because they can irritate the scalp. The "carrier" oil is normally almond or wheat germ oil, but sunflower or simple vegetable cooking oil may be used instead. You may also use infused oil, such as comfrey or St. John's wort. Basic oils quickly deteriorate until diluted, so prepare mixtures as required. A 5% solution of essential oil in the base is appropriate (e.g., 5 drops to 5 ml of carrier oil). While good massage requires experience and practice, the oils can be used at home for localized issues like aching knees or chesty coughs. Pour 2–5 mL of oil into your hand and gently massage the affected area. Sprains benefit from infused comfrey oil, inflammations from St. John's wort oil, and arthritic conditions from bladderwrack oil.

Creams and Ointments from Infused Oils

To make ointments or creams, both hot and cold flavored oils may be thickened with different fats and waxes, such as beeswax, cocoa butter, shea butter, and anhydrous lanolin.

Medicated ointment: Using 100 mL infused oil, 15 g beeswax, and 20 g cocoa butter to make the candle. In a double saucepan, melt the wax and fat, then pour the flavored oil. While still wet, pour into clean glass jars and set aside to cool.

Cream: Use 100 mL infused milk, 20 g beeswax, 20 g anhydrous lanolin, and 50 mL herbal tincture to make the cream. In a double saucepan, melt the wax and fat, add the flavored oil and whisk until fully melted. Remove from the oven. Warm the tincture to a comparable temperature, then gently pour it into the molten mixture while stirring constantly. Various oil and herb/tincture blends may be used to produce various combination creams, such as comfrey and rosemary for arthritic pain or chamomile and St. John's wort for inflammation.

A Natural Alternative to Emulsifying Ointment

A mixture of organic oils and waxes may be used instead of emulsifying ointment to make the cream. Follow the instructions on p. 146. Instead of the emulsifying ointment, melt 25 g white beeswax and 25 g anhydrous lanolin, add 100 g sunflower oil, 25 ml glycerol, 75 ml water, and 50 g dried herb. As before, heat and pressure, but as a preservative, add 5 drops of benzoin to the cooling mixture.

Steam Inhalants

They are great for nasal inflammation caused by catarrh, asthma, sinusitis, hay fever, or other allergies.

- In a mixing cup, place the herb (usually 1 tablespoon of the dried herb would suffice).
- Fill a large mixing bowl halfway with boiling water and add the herb.
- Inhale for as long as you can stand the sun or before the mixture cools.

- For at least 30 minutes after the inhalation, avoid entering into a cold environment.

Reduced Alcohol Tinctures

A tincture based on ethyl alcohol may not be appropriate in certain situations, such as when treating infants, pregnant women, gastric or liver inflammation, or reformed alcoholics. Adding a small volume (25–50 ml) of almost boiling water to the tincture dosage (usually 5 ml) in a cup and allowing it to cool, much of the alcohol would be effectively evaporated. Alternatively, tinctures may be made with glycerol, wine, or cider vinegar. These are made in the same manner as tinctures made from alcohol. Glycerol has the drawback of being ineffective as a solvent for sticky or resinous herbs that could be incompletely processed. Since vinegar-based tinctures (also known as acetracts) had an acidic flavor, they were usually sweetened with honey to produce an oxymel. Vinegar is an expectorant, and acetracts can be used to treat coughs in some cases. However, since vinegar interacts chemically with certain plant constituents and can cause additional side effects, acetracts may not be used for long periods or significant quantities.

Fluid Extracts

These are manufactured in a commercial setting, which necessitates specialized equipment that is not readily available at home. Since they are more concentrated than tinctures (one-to-one weight-to-volume ratio), they can be used in smaller amounts.

Tonic Wines

This is a fun way to take your medication, particularly if you use roots like he shou wu, dang gui, or ginseng. Put 500 g of the herb in a vat or big jug and cover with 2 liters of high-quality wine (preferably red) to save the herb from becoming moldy. Cover the vat with plastic wrap and set it aside for at least two weeks. Take a single dosage the size of a sherry bottle.

Macerations

Some plants, such as marshmallow and valerian seeds, are better macerated than flavored or decocted and then used in the same manner.

Pour 500 mL of water over 30 g of dried root and leave to soak overnight in a cool spot. Until using, strain.

Chinese Decoctions

Herbs are commonly consumed in China as decoctions or soups (teng). Up to 150 g of dried herb in 1 liter of water is decreased to 300–400 ml for three doses, far higher than in the West. The resulting mixture is extremely concentrated, and it might be necessary to dilute it with water to satisfy Western tastes.

Lotions

A lotion is a water-based solution added to the skin to provide relaxing or healing relief from itching or inflammation. It may also be used as a dishwashing liquid. To improve the cooling effect, apply alcohol-based mixtures like tinctures to the lotion. For example, a lotion to relieve skin discomfort might contain 40 milliliters of rosewater, 20 milliliters borage juice, 20 milliliters distilled witch hazel, and 20 milliliters chickweed tincture. Two to three times a day, a small amount of the lotion can be added to cotton wool or absorbent gauze. If you are treating a specific local place, it is good to cover it with a bandage afterward.

Washes

Wounds, sores, skin rashes, ulcers, and other wounds should be bathed with infusions or diluted tinctures. Apply the wash bathing with cotton wool from the middle of the cut or sore outwards. A plastic atomizer may be used to spray the paste on rashes or varicose ulcers.

Pessaries and Suppositories

Special molds that can accommodate up to 24 pessaries or suppositories in different sizes are accessible. Cooking foil may be cut into a small sausage shape (about 1 cm in diameter and 2 cm long) or molded over a thimble to make homemade molds. To begin, lubricate the molds by pouring a small amount of lubricant into each one (made from a mixture of 20 ml soft soap, 100 ml glycerin, and 80 ml of industrial alcohol or methylated spirits). Pour out the lubricant for a few minutes, then drink the alcohol or methylated spirits). Pour off the lubricant after a few minutes, drain properly, and then fill with the pessary mixture. In a double saucepan, melt 20 g cocoa butter and then stir in 10–20 drops (0.5–1 ml) essential oil. You should keep the leftover pessary lubricant in a clean glass container for later use. Alternatively, combine 15 g gelatin with 20 g glycerin, and 30 ml diluted herb infusions or tinctures. Open the mold after it has been set (about 2 hours) and remove the pessaries, which should be kept in a cool spot.

Juices

Herb juices can be produced by pulping the herb in a home juicer or food processor. To get the juice, squeeze the mixture into a jelly bag. Herbs in large quantities are needed (a 2-gallon bucket full of fresh herbs may yield only 100 ml or less juice).

Herbal First Aid

We are more likely to opt for the traditional over-the-counter medications that fill the typical first aid box in a domestic emergency than to resort to natural medicines. On the other hand, herbs may be useful solutions to certain pharmacy offerings. They could be used where a regular first-aid package is not, such as using yarrow to avoid a spontaneous nosebleed in the middle of nowhere. To substitute fresh alternatives at home, a variety of patented herbal formulations are available.

Remedies to Buy

Creams, natural oils, flower treatments, and capsules are just a few of the herbal remedies that are accessible. Here are a few of the most useful herbal medicines to have in your first aid kit at home.

Arnica Tablets (6x)

For any domestic surprises or injuries, this is a must-have. The tablets should be taken every 30 minutes until the patient is more at ease.

Rescue Remedy

The Bach Flower Remedies have a strong emotional effect. Shocks and nervous upsets benefit from Rescue Remedy (also available as a cream).

Arnica Cream

It is great for fractures and sprains, but avoid using it on cracked skin because it will irritate it. A compress soaked in arnica tincture – 1 teaspoon to 500 ml of water – is another choice.

Comfrey Ointment

This promotes cell formation, which speeds up the healing process. Just use it on clean wounds, as the fast healing may trap dirt in the wound. Otherwise, the wound's rapid healing may trap dirt.

Marigold Cream

Calendula is a common name for this flower. This antiseptic and antifungal cream should be used to treat athlete's foot or thrush, as well as bruises, grazes, and dry skin or eczema spots.

Chickweed Cream

Traditionally used to treat eczema and useful for wounds, scalds, and drawing ointment for extracting contaminants from boils and abscesses, bee stings, and stubborn splinters.

Tea Tree Oil

For wounds, grazes, and other skin diseases, this is extremely antiseptic and antifungal. Vaginal thrush should be treated with a cream. On warts and cold sores, a few drops of the oil should be used directly.

Lavender Oil

At the slightest sign of a fever or migraine, mix 2–3 drops in a teaspoon of vegetable oil and rub onto the nape of the neck and temples. Soothe mild wounds, scalds, sunburns, and cold sores in the same mixture.

Thyme Oil

Coughs and chesty colds should be treated with 2–3 drops in a teaspoon of vegetable oil as a chest rub.

Evening Primrose Capsules

These can be used to treat a hangover. The "morning after," a high dose (2–3 g) provides immediate relief.

Distilled Witch Hazel

While a swab soaked in distilled witch-hazel staunches blood flow from cuts, eases varicose veins, and soothes bug bites, this may be used for mild burns and sunburn. Hold an ice cube tray with distilled witch-hazel in the fridge for injuries and sprains – adding, of necessity, that they are specifically labeled!

Syrup

Look for thyme and licorice, horehound and aniseed, or blends containing mousear, hyssop, elecampane, or Iceland moss among the many patent herbal cough syrups available.

Homemade Remedies

Many of the most useful first aid treatments are raw ingredients found in the kitchen cupboard, such as garlic, ginger, and herbal teas. Infused oils can also be produced while the plants are in season and used all year long.

Infused Oils

St. John's wort oil is good for burns and sunburns; marigold oil is good for fungal infections (like athlete's foot), dry skin, and grazes; comfrey oil is good for bruises, sprains, or arthritic joints; rosemary oil is good for rheumatic aches and pains, and lemon balm oil is good for insect bites and insect repellent.

Garlic

Use smashed garlic to draw corns or brush the intensely antiseptic cloves on acne pustules and other contaminated areas.

Honey

Runny honey may be used to dry wounds or to remove pus from contaminated cuts.

Dried Herbs

Using chamomile flowers as a steam inhalation (1 tablespoon of flowers in a big basin of boiling water) for catarrh, hay fever, or moderate asthma attacks, or drink as an infusion for shock and nervous upsets. For oral ulcers and sore throats, use a good infusion of sage as a mouthwash or gargle. Fennel or peppermint tea can help with indigestion, elderflower tea can help with colds and catarrh, and lavender tea can help with headaches.

Aloe

Break off a leaf from an Aloe vera vine, slice it open, and add the dense sap to the infected region right away to soothe mild wounds, scalds, or sunburn.

Ginger

To relieve chills, make a decoction of fresh root with a touch of ground cinnamon, or chew crystallized ginger or ginger cookies.

Onions

New slices should be used to treat bee stings. Cough syrup can be made at home by layering onion slices with brown sugar or honey overnight, collecting the thick brown syrup, and taking 5–10 ml three or four times daily as required.

In The Field

In a rural disaster, search for yarrow for cuts and nosebleeds, crushed daisies for fractures and sprains, shepherd's purse, self-heal, woundwort, wild geranium, or herb Robert to stop bleeding, and shepherd's purse, self-heal, woundwort, wild geranium, or herb Robert to stop bleeding. For bee bites, use new plantain or lemon balm and dock leaves for nettle stings.

Easy to Prepare Home Remedies

Herbalism has long been thought of as "people's medicine" – basic home remedies that can be used with various mild ailments or complement more potent remedies recommended by physicians for chronic and severe disorders. Herbs can be consumed simply as teas, but more sophisticated formulations can be made at home or purchased as patent medicines from health food stores and pharmacies. Even though most herbs are inherently harmless, they must be handled with caution. If symptoms remain, intensify, or the true diagnosis is in question, do not exceed specified doses or proceed with home remedies.

How to Use This Section

Ailments are organized in this segment by body processes, life cycles, or intervention. While herbs can be used for far more illnesses than those mentioned here, the symptoms addressed are those where home remedies are most suitable. The list of complaints is not meant to be extensive or exhaustive, and the herbs mentioned for each ailment are just a small sample of the several plants that may be appropriate in each case. Individual treatments are always chosen based on supply; however, while choosing herbs for specific illnesses, use those who tend to provide the more appropriate behavior for the situation. Do you need an expectorant to remove phlegm, a suppressant to relieve a constant annoying tickle, an antibacterial to fight infection, or a tonic to improve weak lungs, for example, if you have a cough?

Herbs can be very effective quickly, particularly in emergency situations. On the other hand, long-term, persistent illnesses can necessitate therapy for several months before seeing meaningful results. It was once believed that one needed to take a cure for one month for a year that an illness existed. Cyclical disorders, such as menstrual irregularities, usually recover in two to three months. Symptoms can usually improve as the week passes, so be willing to revisit the remedy at least once a month and make adjustments to accommodate new circumstances. Professional herbalists can usually switch medications every few weeks when wellbeing and energy levels fluctuate.

Consult a nurse whether you have an ailment that is not covered in this segment or if you have a chronic illness. If you collect herbs in the wild or from gardens, consult a good plant key or field herbal to make sure you pick the right plants for the job.

Cautions

- If an acute illness – fevers, coughs, stomach upsets, intense headaches, etc. – does not improve after a few days or seems to be deteriorating, seek immediate attention.
- If you are taking medicine for a certain ailment, please check with your doctor or another care provider before adjusting your dose. Since certain herbs interfere with conventional medications, caution is advised in some cases.

- Based on their age, children should receive a percentage of the maximum adult dosage.
- Since metabolism speeds down as people age, normal adult doses can be lowered as frailty and weight loss increase.
- Essential oils are highly concentrated, and many of them can irritate mucous membranes. Do not take essential oils internally under competent medical supervision as otherwise specified in the remedy charts. Dilute essential oils in a carrier oil before applying to the skin – wheatgerm, almond, or avocado are the safest. Still, sunflower, olive, or safflower will do if that is all you have. Due to the high cost of natural oils, many industrial chemical alternatives are available for purchase. Do not be fooled by low-cost products; only buy a reputable brand guaranteed to be genuine and unadulterated.

Aches & Pains

The typical response to muscle pain is to search for painkillers such as aspirin, paracetamol, or codeine, which rapidly lull the body back into pain-free bliss. Pain, on the other hand, is just a symptom, a signal that everything is not quite right. Pulled muscles and torn tendons need little mobility to heal, and those annoying twinges urge us to relax as much as possible while the body recovers.

Many plants function as muscle relaxants and antispasmodics, anti-inflammatories, and cell proliferates, reversing the damage caused by physical injuries or degenerative diseases like osteoarthritis. For muscle or joint pain, essential oils may be the most powerful. When massaged into arthritic joints or used on hot compresses, diluted rosemary essence will provide immediate symptomatic relief.

While symptomatic relief is important, it does not always solve the problem: an herbal approach to osteoarthritis might include comfrey ointment to encourage the repair of damaged and degenerating bone, anti-inflammatory herbs like willow, devil's claw, or meadowsweet to help relieve pain, and cleansing plants like yellow dock, burdock, or celery seed to help the body rid itself of toxins.

Arthritis and rheumatic pains are referred to as "bi syndrome" in traditional Chinese medicine and are blamed on the same "external evils" – wind, damp, cold, or heat – that trigger colds and fevers. Warming diaphoretic herbs like ma huang or gui zhi can cure a "cold" form of the bi syndrome. In contrast, others, like bai zhu or bai Shao Yao, can be used to boost the body's essential energies and increase qi circulation, helping to deter further attacks by other "evils."

Sprains and Strains

Accidental joint and muscle fractures, including back strains. If you believe or know you have an injury, or if your symptoms have not improved after a few days, seek immediate medical attention.

Key Symptoms

- Pain following obvious injury or exertion.
- Swollen joints or limbs.
- Bruising.

Remedies

1. Arnica Montana—**ARNICA**

Flowers

- Actions: Wound herb and antibacterial, causes reabsorption of internal bleeding for bruises and sprains.
- How to use: Externally use cream or dilute tincture as a compress; take Arnica 6X every 1–2 hours.
- Combinations: Use as a simple.
- Precautions: Do not use on broken skin; only take homeopathic arnica internally.

2. Symphytum officinale—**COMFREY**

Infused Oil

- Actions: Encourages cell growth of connective tissues and bones; breaks down red blood cells in bruising.
- How to use: Use an ointment or infused oil frequently as required.

- Combinations: Add 5–10 drops of essential oils, such as thyme, lavender, or juniper, to 25 ml infused oil.
- Precautions: Only use if the injury is clean; not advisable for long-term internal use.

3. Thymus vulgaris—**THYME**

Essential Oil

- Actions: Antispasmodic and stimulant encouraging blood flow to the tissue to encourage repair.
- How to use: Use 10 drops of oil to 25 ml water in a compress, or 10 drops in a hot bath.
- Combinations: Other essential oils, such as lavender, rosemary, or sage, in an almond or sunflower base as a massage oil.
- Precautions: Massage can be damaging if given too soon after injury.

Arthritis and Rheumatism

Osteoarthritis (OA) is caused by joint wear and tear, but it can also be caused by cold and humid conditions. Rheumatoid arthritis (RA) is a disease that causes inflammation in many joints, normally symmetrically, and necessitates medical attention. Rheumatism refers to any muscle or joint pain, while lumbago is a term for low back pain.

Key Symptoms

- Stiffness and joint pain.
- Creaking sounds in joints.
- Joint deformities and swellings.
- Joints may feel hot or burning in RA.
- Symmetric joint swellings in RA.
- Symptoms are often worse in damp weather in OA.
- Frozen shoulder (chronic stiffness and pain in the shoulder joint) can be treated as OA.

Remedies

1. Harpagophytum procumbens—**DEVIL'S CLAW**

Root

- Actions: Potent anti-inflammatory; action has been compared with cortisone. Better for OA and degenerative conditions.
- How to use: Use 1–3 g powder daily in capsule form in the acute phase; up to 15 ml tincture daily or in combinations.
- Combinations: Often taken as simple but can be combined with tinctures of angelica, St. John's wort, bogbean, or celery seed.

2. Salix alba—**WILLOW**

Bark

- Actions: Rich in salicylates, which are anti-inflammatory and cooling for hot joints; useful in acute phases.
- How to use: Up to 5 ml of the fluid extract three times daily or with other tinctures in combinations.

- Combinations: Can be used with tinctures of angelica, black cohosh, lignum vitae, yellow dock, or burdock.
- Precautions: Avoid in cases of salicylate allergy.

3. Menyanthes trifoliata—**BOGBEAN**

Leaves

- Actions: Cleansing, cooling, and anti-inflammatory: a useful herb for "hotter" types of arthritis and muscle pain.
- How to use: Up to 8 ml of the tincture three times daily; also as an infusion or macerate 10 g in 100 ml red wine.
- Combinations: In decoctions with black cohosh or celery seeds; in tinctures with St. John's wort, meadowsweet, or prickly ash bark.

4. Angelica archangelica—**ANGELICA**

Root

- Actions: Good for "cold" type arthritis: warming and stimulating.

- How to use: Dilute tincture or infusion as a compressor internally as a standard decoction.
- Combinations: Add celery seed or prickly ash to decoctions.
- Precautions: Avoid pregnancy.

Gout

Generally associated with the buildup of uric acid in joints, it may be linked to dietary excess.

Key Symptoms

- Swollen, inflamed, and very painful joints.
- Toes or foot joints are often affected.

Remedies

1. Apium graveolens—**CELERY**

Seed

- Actions: Clears uric acid from joints; useful in both gout and arthritic problems.
- How to use: In infusions (1 teaspoon to 500 ml water) or combined with other tinctures.
- Combinations: With lignum vitae in infusions; tincture with yarrow, gravel root, or burdock.
- Precautions: Use only seeds intended for medicinal use; avoid in pregnancy.

2. Teucrium chamaedrys—**WALL GERMANDER**

Aerial Parts

- Actions: Bitter digestive tonic and diuretic.
- How to use: Standard infusion or up to 15 ml of tincture daily.
- Combinations: Combine with yarrow and celery seed in infusions or with burdock and gravel root in tincture.

Rheumatism or Myalgia

Rheumatism is a broad word that refers to a variety of muscle aches and pains (myalgia). It could be due to fibrositis (muscle and muscle sheath inflammation), mostly affecting the back, or simply due to overexertion.

Key Symptoms

- Painful, sore, aching muscles.
- It may be associated with traumatic injury or food intolerance.

Remedies

1. Actaea racemosa—**BLACK COHOSH**

Root

- Actions: Analgesic, cooling, and soothing; contains salicylic acid to reduce inflammation and ease stiffness.

- How to use: Take a decoction or 10–40 drops of tincture per dose, three times daily; take 1 x 200 mg capsule up to three times a day.
- Combinations: Combine with bogbean in decoctions or anti-inflammatories like devil's claw in capsules.

2. Rosmarinus officinalis—**ROSEMARY**

Essential Oil

- Actions: Stimulating, analgesic, and antirheumatic; warms muscles by encouraging blood flow to the area.
- How to use: Use 10 drops of oil in 5 ml of infused bladderwrack oil as a massage as required. Also helpful for arthritic pains.
- Combinations: Use infused St. John's wort as an alternative base or add additional warming and analgesic essential oils such as eucalyptus, juniper, hyssop, or thyme.

Backache & Lumbago

Backache is a common ailment caused by pulled muscles, broken discs, nerve injuries, strains, or kidney weakness. Lumbago is a term used to describe low back pain in the lumbar region.

Key Symptoms

- Pain can be chronic, debilitating, and restrict movement.

Important: Seek professional help for any persistent back pain of unknown cause.

Remedies

1. Berberis vulgaris—**BARBERRY**

Stem Bark

- Actions: Anti-inflammatory, cleansing can be especially helpful for low back pains.
- How to use: Take in decoction, half a cup per dose, or up to 5 ml of tincture, three times daily.

- Combinations: With diuretics like celery seed, buchu, and horsetail for back pain associated with kidney problems; with anti-inflammatories, such as black cohosh and devil's claw for muscle or joint inflammations.
- Precautions: Avoid pregnancy.

2. Juniperis communis—**JUNIPER**

Berries & Essential Oil

- Actions: Antirheumatic, stimulating, clear excess lactic acid from muscles.
- How to use: Take 10–20 drops of tincture per dose; use half a teaspoon of crushed berries per cup of infusion; use 10 drops of essential oil per 5 ml almond oil as external massage.
- Combinations: Use analgesics and anti-inflammatories such as valerian, devil's claw, white willow, and black cohosh in tinctures or capsules (2 x 200 mg capsules per dose).
- Precautions: Avoid in pregnancy; do not take internally for longer than six weeks without a break; do not take if there is any kidney damage or disease.

Tennis Elbow & Tenosynovitis

Tenosynovitis is an inflammation of the tendon sheaths that typically affects the hand, forearm, or fingertips. Simultaneously, tennis or golfer's elbow is an inflammation of the bursa – a thin sac filled with fluid that is part of the joint.

Key Symptoms

- Pain and difficulty in moving the affected joint.
- Numbness or tingling in the fingers.
- Worse when twisting the joint.

Remedies

1. Guaiacum officinalis—**LIGNUM VITAE**

Heartwood

- Actions: Anti-inflammatory and cooling suitable for any muscle or joint inflammations, including tendon problems.

- How to use: Take half a cup of decoction made from half a teaspoon of chippings per cup; take up to 10 ml of tincture per day.
- Combinations: Antispasmodics and anti-inflammatories like guelder rose, prickly ash bark, and black cohosh in tinctures or decoctions.

2. Achillea millefolium—**YARROW**

Aerial Parts & Essential Oil

- Actions: Reduces inflammation in joints, tendons, and muscles to give pain relief and improve movement.
- How to use: Use 10 drops of essential oil in 20 ml of infused St. John's wort oil as a massage; use a cold, chilled infusion for soaking a compress to relieve pain and stiffness.
- Combinations: Use lavender oil in external massage or combine with stinging nettle and arnica infusions in a compress.
- Precautions: Prolonged use may cause skin rashes or increase photosensitivity in rare cases.

Repetitive Strain Injury (RSI)

Spasms and fatigue in the hands, head, shoulders, spine, or back are caused by repeated physical movements that cause tissue loss over time.

Key Symptoms

- Extreme pain in moving or manipulating the limbs or fingers.
- Sudden onset may be preceded by numbness and tingling.
- Limbs may be extremely sensitive and excruciating to touch.

Remedies

1. Lentinus edodes—**SHIITAKE**

Mushrooms

- Actions: Tonics like shiitake can help to improve the body's ability to cope with physical stress while reducing the inflammation associated with the symptoms.

- How to use: Take up to 10 g of dried shiitake powder per dose with water; decoction use 90 g of fresh mushrooms in a daily soup.
- Combinations: Add Siberian ginseng or huang qi powders, or add a piece of either root to the soup and simmer for at least 50 minutes to increase resistance to stress and tonify the system.

2. Filipendula ulmaria—**MEADOWSWEET**

Aerial Parts

- Actions: Contains salicylates to reduce inflammation and ease pain; gentle digestive stimulate to improve metabolism.
- How to use: Use in infusion or tincture.
- Combinations: With nervines such as St. John's wort and vervain in infusions; with white willow and valerian in tinctures.
- Precautions: Avoid in cases of salicylate allergy.

Sciatica

The sciatic nerve, which stretches from the spine across the back and outer thigh to the foot, is irritated or compressed, resulting in nerve pain. Disc loss is a common cause. The term is used to describe some kind of backache, but it can only describe complications involving the sciatic nerve.

Key Symptoms

- Back pain and stiffness; pain travels along the path of the nerve.
- Pain on bending or picking up items from the floor.

Remedies

1. Zanthoxylum americanum—**PRICKLY ASH**

Bark

- Actions: Stimulates circulation to supply nutrients to tissue and help repair and remove wastes; eases spasmodic pains.

- How to use: Use in decoctions (half a teaspoon per cup) or take up to 10 ml of tincture daily.
- Combinations: In decoctions with anti-inflammatories and nervines such as lignum vitae, black cohosh, and valerian; in tinctures with St. John's wort, white willow, and black cohosh.

2. Capsicum frutescens—**CAYENNE**

Fruit

- Actions: Stimulates blood flow, strengthens the nerves, and relieves nerve pains.
- How to use: Use the infused oil in massage or take 5 drops of tincture in water per dose.
- Combinations: Add 2–5 drops of juniper or rosemary oil to the infused oil as additional circulatory stimulants; add up to 5 ml of nervines like St. John's wort or valerian tincture per dose.
- Precautions: Prolonged or excessive topical use may lead to blistering.

Cramp

Muscle spasms can be debilitating and last for a long time. It may be linked to a salt deficiency, as well as stress and exhaustion.

Key Symptoms

- Sharp, severe pain in the legs.
- Affected muscle feels hard and rigid to touch.

Remedies

1. Viburnum opulus —**GUELDER ROSE**

Bark

- Action: Effective relaxant for both smooth and skeletal muscle; anti-inflammatory.
- How to use: Use 25% tincture in rosewater as a lotion or in creams.
- Combinations: Combines well with Indian tobacco in cramp creams.

2. Dioscorea villosa—**WILD YAM**

Rhizome

- Action: Muscle relaxant and mild peripheral vasodilator.
- How to use: Sip a standard decoction or take 20 drops of tincture and repeat every 15 minutes if symptoms persist.
- Combinations: As a simple or with guelder rose tincture.
- Precautions: Avoid pregnancy unless under professional guidance.

Headaches & Migraines

Headaches and migraines should be seen as signs of a disorder rather than distinct diseases, and a systematic approach to health care often searches at the root sources of pain. Of course, headaches may be linked to stress or tension; soothing, sedating herbs (known as nervines) can be beneficial. Chronic stress headaches may indicate a need for a complete lifestyle overhaul or simply a need to learn simple coping strategies to cope with everyday pressures. Head pain may be caused by nasal catarrh and sinusitis, which normally occurs in the frontal sinuses, above the nose, and below the eyes. Elderflower, marshmallow root, golden pine, hyssop, or bistort are all decongestant herbs used to clear the upper respiratory tract. Fresh air and a diet low in mucus-forming ingredients (dairy, alcohol, and sugars, and processed carbohydrates) will also aid.

Migraines are headaches caused by optical hallucinations such as blinking lights that zigzag around the visual field, and they can be caused by food intolerance or pollutants. Some migraines are "hot," and ice packs can help, while others are "cold," and a hot towel on the forehead can help. Soothing, calming herbs like rosemary, ginger, or gui zhi work best for "cold" migraines, while refreshing, bitter herbs like lavender and vervain work best for "hot" migraines. In traditional Chinese medicine, the eyes are closely associated with liver activity, and migraines, with their vision disturbances and light exposure, can be diagnosed with over-exuberant liver qi or pathogenic "wind" influencing the liver.

Important Note: If you have sudden recurring headaches or notice a difference in the pattern of your daily headaches, see a doctor.

Tension Headaches

Tightening of the neck muscles because of tension or anxiety can be the cause. Relaxation can help to alleviate symptoms.

Key Symptoms

- Pain, generally frontal.

REMEDIES

1. Stachys officinalis—**WOOD BETONY**

Aerial Parts

- Actions: Sedative and stimulant for cerebral circulation; useful nervine for anxiety and worries.
- How to use: Standard infusion or tincture.
- Combination: Add lavender, vervain, St. John's wort, skullcap to infusion or tincture.
- Precautions: Avoid high doses in pregnancy.

2. Scutellaria lateriflora—**SKULLCAP**

Aerial Parts

- Actions: Relaxant and restorative for the central nervous system; sedative and antispasmodic.
- How to use: Standard infusion or tincture.
- Combination: Mix 45 ml of skullcap tincture and 5 ml of lemon balm and take 5 ml doses (up to four times daily).

Migraine

It may be due to insulin allergy, the menstrual cycle, or other sources of stress. It is linked to improvements in the stress in the brain's arteries. Symptoms that go untreated will last anywhere from a few minutes to several days.

Key Symptoms

- Characteristic visual disturbances always precede pain.
- Pins and needles in limbs.
- Sickness and nausea.
- Light sensitivity.

Remedies

1. Tanacetum parthenium—**FEVERFEW**

Aerial Parts

- Actions: Anti-inflammatory, dilates cerebral blood vessels so helpful for migraines associated with constriction.
- How to use: Eat one leaf daily as a prophylactic or use 10 drops of tincture every 30 minutes while symptoms persist.
- Combination: Combine with valerian or Jamaican dogwood tincture in drop doses.
- Precautions: Side-effects can include mouth ulceration; avoid if taking anticoagulant drugs such as warfarin.

2. Lavandula spp.—**LAVENDER**

Flowers & Essential Oil

- Actions: Sedative and analgesic with antispasmodic action.
- How to use: Massage lavender oil (neat or diluted 50:50 with a carrier oil) into temples at the first hint of symptoms.

- Combination: Follow massage treatment by drinking lavender flower and vervain infusion.
- Precautions: Do not take lavender oil internally without professional guidance.

3. Gelsemium Sempervirens—**YELLOW JASMINE**

Root

- Actions: Potent analgesic and sedative that can be used for migraine and neuralgia.
- How to use: 5 drops of 1:10 tincture in water; repeat up to four times daily while pain persists. Maximum dose 5 ml per week.
- Combination: Best as simple in the acute phase; can combine with Jamaican dogwood or lavender.
- Precautions: Use is restricted to professional practitioners in some geographies. Overdose can cause nausea and double vision.

Facial or Trigeminal Neuralgia

The facial or trigeminal nerves are often followed by severe burning and stabbing pain. It may occur as a result of an illness or exposure to frost and draughts.

KEY SYMPTOMS

- Very localized pain that is severe.
- Related skin areas are highly sensitive to touch.
- May recur regularly.

REMEDIES: Citrus x Limon—LEMON

FRUIT & ESSENTIAL OIL

- Actions: Cooling, astringent, reputed nerve tonic, and anti-inflammatory
- Combinations: Gently rub a slice of fresh lemon or a little juice on the affected area, or use well-diluted lemon oil.
- How to use: Use as a simple for symptomatic relief.

- Precautions: Lemon oil can be irritant; use no more than 5 drops in 25 ml of carrier oil.

1. Hypericum perforatum—**ST. JOHN'S WORT**

Aerial Parts

- Actions: Trophorestorative for the nervous system and anti-inflammatory.
- Combinations: Standard infusion internally plus infused oil applied externally to the affected area.
- How to use: Add lavender and skullcap to infusion.
- Precautions: Avoid internal use if taking prescription medicine; seek professional advice.

2. Verbena officinalis—**VERVAIN**

Aerial Parts

- Actions: Sedative, antispasmodic and restorative for the nervous system.

- How to use: Use as a poultice of fresh leaves or an infusion as a compress on the affected area and take the standard infusion or tincture internally.
- Combinations: Add lavender or St. John's wort to tincture or infusion or up to 20 drops of Jamaican dogwood tincture.
- Precautions: Avoid high doses in pregnancy.

Infections

Infections are now attributed to a variety of bacteria and viruses; prior centuries blamed "flying venom," "elf-shot," or the "evil eye," while Chinese medicine blames the "six evils" (wind, frost, heat, dampness, dryness, and fire) for certain chills and fevers, with "pestilence" to blame for serious epidemics. Many of the plants used to treat various ailments have now been discovered to be powerful antibiotics and immune system stimulants. The Chinese tonic herb huang qi, for example, is used to enhance the wei qi, or defensive force, which defends the exterior of the body from attack by those six evils. It is now classified as both an antibacterial and an immunostimulant. It inhibits the development of

Streptococci, Staphylococci, and other bacteria and increases the body's generation of macrophages (scavenger cells that eat attacking bacteria), and generally enhancing protection mechanisms. These antibacterial herbs, unlike wide-spectrum antibiotics, appear to be unique to the species that they destroy, meaning they have fewer effects on the helpful bacteria that live in our guts, and hence the intestinal upsets that may accompany orthodox medicine are less probable.

Herbs may also be used to manage the progression of an infection as the body attempts to rebalance itself. Colds can be either "hot" or "cold" in nature, and they can alternate between the two as the disease progresses. Warming herbs such as ginger, gui zhi, or angelica are required in “cold” conditions. Diaphoretics and the many febrifuges that once played an important role in fever control will help cool “hot” infections: Consider herbs like boneset, catmint, peppermint, or mulberry leaf.

Colds and Flu

While often associated with external pressures, fatigue, depression, excessive cold, or heat, it is generally thought to be caused by bacterial or viral infections.

Key Symptoms

- Fever.
- Muscle pain and/or headache.
- Nasal catarrh, stuffiness.
- Coughs.
- Sore throat.

Remedies

1. Eupatorium perfoliatum—**BONESET**

Aerial Parts

- Actions: Diaphoretic, febrifuge, and expectorant useful in hot, feverish colds and flu with joint or muscle pain.

- How to use: Standard dose of infusion or tincture 3–4 times daily.
- Combinations: Use with an arrow, elderflowers, and peppermint in flu and feverish colds.
- Precautions: High doses are emetic.

2. Allium sativa—**GARLIC**

Clove

- Actions: Effective antimicrobial and antifungal suitable for a wide range of infectious conditions.
- How to use: Up to 5 fresh cloves daily in acute conditions, or use prepared capsules.
- Combinations: Best as simple. Eat parsley if concerned about garlic smells.
- Precautions: Can be stomach irritant; if so, use ginger or fennel tea to reduce symptoms. Avoid therapeutic doses in pregnancy/lactation.

3. Nepeta cataria—**CATMINT**

Aerial Parts

- Actions: Cooling in fevers encourages sweating and is astringent in catarrhal congestion.
- How to use: Standard dose of infusion or tincture 3–4 times daily.
- Combinations: For feverish colds, add yarrow, elderflower, boneset, ground ivy, or mulberry leaf.

4. Cinnamomum cassia—**CINNAMON**

Twigs

- Actions: Warming for cold conditions, diaphoretic with antibacterial action.
- How to use: Standard decoction or tincture; use cinnamon bark if twigs unavailable.
- Combinations: With fresh ginger root in chills.
- Precautions: Avoid pregnancy. Not suitable for hot, feverish colds.

Boils and Abscesses

Staphylococcus aureus penetrating the hair follicle or an infected wound is the most common cause of localized infection. This is a sign of a compromised immune system.

Key Symptoms

- Tender, inflamed area of skin – although abscesses may be found in other parts of the body.
- Boils contain obvious pus, which may need a surgical incision.
- It can be painful.

Remedies

1. Forsythia suspensa—**LIAN QIAO**

Berries

- Actions: Broad-spectrum antibacterial, anti-inflammatory, and antipyretic to resolve abscesses and boils; also for fevers.
- How to use: Standard decoction.
- Combinations: Combine with honeysuckle flowers, burdock seeds, or huang qin, and take echinacea in capsules.

- Precautions: Use before boils start to suppurate; Avoid diarrhea.

2. Scrophularia spp.—**FIGWORT**

Aerial Parts and Xuan Shen Root

- Actions: Anti-inflammatory and antibacterial. Cleansing herbs for toxic conditions.
- How to use: Use figwort leaves as a poultice; take a standard decoction or tincture of xuan shen.
- Combinations: Add lian qiao, honeysuckle flowers, goldenseal, huang qin, or echinacea to the decoction.
- Precautions: Heart stimulant – avoid heartbeat abnormalities (tachycardia).

Immune Stimulants

A weakened immune system can be linked to fatigue, depression, or a more severe underlying disease.

Key Symptoms

- Persistent colds or flu.
- Regular fungal or skin infections.
- Chronic fatigue.

Remedies

1. Astragalus membranaceus—**HUANG QI RHIZOME**
    - Actions: Increases production of white blood cells and strengthens immune response; also antibacterial and energy tonic.
    - How to use: Standard decoction or tincture.
    - Combinations: With other energy tonics – licorice, dang gui, bai zhu in debilitated conditions.
    - Precautions: Avoid if the condition involves excess heat or yin deficiency.
2. Echinacea spp.—**ECHINACEA**

Root or Leaves

- Actions: Important antibacterial and antiviral, also strengthens resistance to infections; for all septic or infectious conditions.
- How to use: Take 500 mg of powdered root in capsules or 10 ml of the tincture. Repeat up to four times daily.
- Combinations: Effective as a simple or add elderflower, yarrow, or catmint tinctures.

Respiratory Problems

A holistic approach to wellness demands that sickness be addressed not only on a physical basis but also on a mental and moral level. Infection, toxic waste, or a failing heart are just a part of the equation for chest problems. The lung is synonymous with the emotion mourning in Chinese medicine, and chest symptoms may also accompany a bereavement or other sorrow; chesty colds, bronchitis, and other obvious "infections" can often strike while we are down – in a job we do not want, depressed at home, or at family distress points. Herbs can not make these problems go away, but lung tonics like elecampane or cowslip, which often have a nervous system effect, can help.

Breathing has a deeper meaning than just taking in oxygen. Prana is the life force of Ayurvedic medicine, and breath control (pranayama) is an important Yogic practice. Breath regulation improves stamina and strength, as well as becoming a calming aid for lung healing. Inflammatory lung symptoms are said to be helped through breathing in through the left nostril and out through the right, whereas cool, damp illnesses are said to be helped through the reverse routine.

Breath is also associated with essential energy in Chinese medicine, and it regulates the flow of qi. The Chinese version of pranayama is qi gong, which is taught to critically ill patients in Chinese hospitals with remarkable success. Breathing disorders are thought to be harmful to critical resources and a symptom of qi weakness or imbalance. Asthma, for example, is said to be caused by a loss of kidney capacity, which interferes with the kidney's ability to pull qi downwards as part of the inhalation process, so care depends on herbs that reinforce the kidney rather than only lung remedies.

Important Note: If you have a recurring cough that you do not know what is causing, you should still seek professional support. Until discontinuing orthodox asthma therapy, chronic asthmatics should seek expert advice.

Coughs

Inflammation or blockage of the bronchial tubes causes this reaction.

Key Symptoms

- A productive cough may vary from thin watery mucous to thick yellow or green phlegm.
- Unproductive cough can be very dry and irritating.
- Often associated with infections – such as colds and influenza.
- It may be associated with nervous tension and without pathological cause.

NB: Always seek professional help for any persistent cough of unknown cause.

Remedies

1. Althaea Officinalis—**MARSHMALLOW**

Leaf or Flower

- Actions: Demulcent and expectorant; soothing for inflamed respiratory mucosa.
- How to use: Standard infusion or tincture; syrup of leaves or flowers in 5 ml dose.
- Combinations: Combine with anti-catarrhals such as ground ivy or additional expectorants such as licorice, mulberry bark, or white horehound.

2. Hyssopus officinalis—**HYSSOP**

Aerial Parts or Essential Oil

- Actions: Warming and expectorant, antispasmodic helpful for bronchitis; also useful for thin, watery phlegm.
- How to use: Standard infusion or tincture; essential oil in chest rubs (5 ml to 20 ml carrier oil).
- Combinations: Can be combined with restoratives such as elecampane and white horehound in chronic conditions. Use 2 parts hyssop to 1 part of the other herb.

- Precautions: Do not take essential oils internally.

3. Morus alba—**MULBERRY (Sang Bai Pi)**

Bark

- Actions: Cooling expectorant and antitussive – good for "hot" conditions.
- How to use: Standard decoction or tincture.
- Combinations: Combine with other soothing or cooling herbs such as marshmallow leaf, ribwort plantain, or thyme if there is an infection.

4. Phyllostachys nigra—**ZHU LI**

Sap or Zhu Ru/Vamsha Rochana Shaving

- Actions: Antimicrobial, cooling, and expectorant to clear the thick, infected yellow sputum or productive coughs.
- How to use: Use 1 teaspoon of shavings per dose in decoctions; 250 mg in capsules or up to 50 drops of tincture; use 5 ml of the fresh sap diluted in water.

- Combinations: Add an equal amount of ginger juice to the sap; add cinnamon, cardamom, or black pepper to the powdered shavings with an equal amount of sugar or honey and take in teaspoon doses. Combine zhu ru with elecampane and ginger in decoctions.
- Precautions: Avoid diarrhea and coughs associated with cold.

5. Prunus serotina—**WILD CHERRY**

Bark

- Actions: Cough suppressant; useful for dry, irritant, or nervous coughs.
- How to use: Standard decoction; 2 ml tincture per dose.
- Combinations: Combine with astringents such as mullein, tonics like elecampane, or additional cough suppressants like wild lettuce.
- Precautions: Suppresses the cough reflex, so it should not be used for productive coughs or infections. It can cause sleepiness.

Catarrh

Excessive mucosal secretions in the lungs. It can be "cold type," with lots of watery secretions, or "hot," with dense, yellow secretions that are difficult to get rid of. Catarrh of the cold type is also linked to sugary snacks and a sluggish system, while catarrh of the hot type is linked to a stressed, anxious disposition.

Key Symptoms

- Post-nasal drip with irritant cough.
- Hot type may involve pain in sinus areas.
- Inflammation of the nasal mucosa.
- It may be associated with colds or allergic conditions.

Remedies

1. Sambucus nigra —**ELDER**

Flowers

- Actions: Anti-catarrhal, anti-inflammatory, and expectorant. For the upper respiratory tract, the catarrh is associated with colds and hay fever.
- How to use: Standard infusion or tincture.
- Combinations: Use other drying and astringent herbs, such as yarrow, ground ivy, goldenrod, agrimony, or bistort.

2. Gnaphalium uliginosum—**MARSH CUDWEED**

Leaves

- Actions: Anti-inflammatory and tonifying to the respiratory mucosa.
- How to use: Standard infusion or tincture.
- Combinations: Use other anti-catarrhal herbs such as elderflowers or goldenrod using 2:1 marsh cudweed to the other herb.

3. Solidago virgaurea—**GOLDEN ROD**

Aerial Parts

- Actions: Drying, astringent, and anti-catarrhal; anti-inflammatory for the mucosa.
- How to use: Standard infusion or tincture.
- Combinations: Can be used with additional anti-catarrhals such as march cudweed, wild indigo, or ribwort plantain.

4. Verbascum Thapsus—**MULLEIN**

Leaves

- Actions: Cooling, astringent, and soothing for thick or hot catarrh and nasal congestion.
- How to use: Take in infusion or tincture.
- Combinations: Combines well with anti-catarrhals like coltsfoot and elderflowers in infusions; add antimicrobials such as thyme or mulberry leaf in infections.

Sinusitis

Inflammation or inflammation affecting the skull's sinus cavities. It may happen after a cold or be linked to dental issues like deep-seated root abscesses.

Key Symptoms

- Generally follows a common cold.
- Pain affecting sinus areas—headaches that can be severe.
- Sinuses tender to the touch.
- Nasal discharge is often streaked with blood.
- Often linked to tense, uptight personality with a tight rein on emotions—unwilling to cry.

Remedies

1. Hydrastis Canadensis—**GOLDENSEAL**

Rhizome

- Actions: Powerful cooling astringent and anti-catarrhal.

- How to use: Use two 200 mg powder in capsules three times daily or 20 drops of tincture per dose.
- Combinations: Add eyebright powder to capsules.
- Precautions: Avoid pregnancy and high blood pressure; do not exceed the stated dose.

2. Myrica cerifera—**BAYBERRY**

Bark

- Actions: Warming and astringent; circulatory stimulant.
- How to use: Use the powder as snuff or add 5 ml tincture to 20 ml emulsifying ointment and use as sinus massage.
- Combinations: Add 2–3 drops of eucalyptus oil to the ointment.
- Precautions: Heating herb so avoids in very "hot" conditions.

3. Glechoma hederacea—**GROUND IVY**

Aerial Parts

- Actions: Anti-catarrhal and astringent suitably drying for catarrh in both sinuses and bronchi.

- How to use: Standard decoction or tincture.
- Combinations: Can be used with other anti-catarrhal herbs such as elderflower, magnolia flowers, ribwort plantain, or yarrow.

4. Piper longum—**PIPPALI/LONG PEPPER**

Fruit

- Actions: Warming anti-catarrhal useful for sinus headaches and also allergic rhinitis.
- How to use: Take in milk infusion, capsules (1–2 times, 200 mg per dose), or up to 40 drops tincture per dose.
- Combinations: Generally used as a simple with milk, but support with antibacterials like thyme, lian qiao, or echinacea in tinctures or capsules where there is infection.

Bronchitis

Bronchitis is an inflammation of the bronchial tubes. It may be acute due to an illness or permanent due to smoking and pollutants.

Key Symptoms

- Productive cough, often purulent sputum.
- Fever, high temperature.
- Chronic bronchitis may involve chest pains and breathlessness and often follows a cold.

Remedies

1. Inula helenium—**ELECAMPANE**

Root

- Action: Lung tonic and expectorant; restorative and warming; good for weakened lungs and old coughs.
- How to use: Standard decoction, tincture, or syrup.
- Combinations: Use as a simple or add 10 ml horsetail juice to heal lung damage, or add hyssop or white horehound to tinctures.

2. Primula veris—**COWSLIP**

Root

- Actions: Potent expectorant good for loosening old phlegm and easing stubborn, dry coughs. Also helpful for asthma.
- How to use: Standard decoction, tincture, or syrup.
- Combinations: Can be combined with other strong expectorants such as gum plant and a soothing demulcent like licorice.

3. Thymus Vulgaris—**THYME**

Aerial Parts Or Essential Oil

- Action: Antiseptic and expectorant; useful for thick, infected phlegm and dry, difficult coughs.
- How to use: Herb in standard infusion syrup or tincture; 10 drops of essential oil in 25 ml almond oil as a chest rub.
- Combinations: Add additional expectorants such as licorice or mulberry bark to syrups and tinctures; add horsetail juice to repair damage or combine the essential oil with hyssop, pine, or peppermint oils in chest rubs.
- Precautions: Do not take essential oils internally.

4. Marrubium vulgare—**WHITE HOREHOUND**

Aerial Parts

- Action: Antispasmodic, demulcent, and expectorant relaxing the bronchi and easing congestion.
- How to use: Standard infusion, tincture, or syrup; horehound candy also available commercially.
- Combinations: Combine with warming expectorants such as hyssop or angelica and tonics like elecampane.

Note: All the herbs listed under bronchitis can also be used in asthmatic conditions.

Asthma

Bronchospasm leading to wheezing and breathlessness.

Key Symptoms

- Characteristic wheeze on expiration.
- It may be associated with other allergic symptoms such as hay fever or eczema.

- It may be a family tendency.
- The great difficulty in breathing.
- It may be associated with fever and infection.

Note: Severe asthma can be life-threatening, and professional medical help may be required.

Remedies

1. Ephedra sinica—**MA HUANG**

Aerail Parts

- Action: Bronchial relaxant and vasodilator; warming for all cold conditions of the chest.
- How to use: 100 mg of dried stems to a cup of water as a decoction or as prescribed. The herb is restricted in some geographies with a maximum dosage in the UK of 2.5 ml of a 1:4 tincture three times daily.

- Combinations: May be prescribed in combination with other herbs such as gum plant, angelica, white horehound, hyssop, or pill-bearing spurge.
- Precautions: Not to be used by patients taking MAO inhibitors as antidepressants; avoid severe hypertension.

2. Matricaria chamomilla—**GERMAN CHAMOMILE**

Flowers

- Action: Anti-allergenic, anti-inflammatory, and antispasmodic – useful for allergic asthma.
- How to use: Use a steam inhalation (1 tablespoon of dried flowers to a bowl of boiling water) at the first sign of an attack. The essential oil can be added to chest rubs and inhalants, Combinations: Support with internal medication as for bronchitis above.

3. Grindelia camporum—**GUMPLANT**

Aerial Parts

- Action: Antispasmodic and expectorant to ease bronchospasm.
- How to use: 15 g herb to 500 ml water for infusions; up to 5 ml daily in doses of 1–2 ml.
- Combinations: Can be combined with additional antispasmodics such as pill-bearing spurge or with expectorants such as cowslip root.
- Precautions: Hypotensive, avoid in cases of low blood pressure. High doses can irritate the kidneys.

4. Eucalyptus globulus—**EUCALYPTUS**

Essential Oil

- Actions: Antiseptic, antispasmodic, and expectorant (also for bronchitis).
- How to use: 40 drops of eucalyptus oil in 20 ml of the carrier as a chest rub; use a few drops on a pillow or handkerchief as an inhalant.
- Combinations: Add a total of 10–15 drops of thyme, peppermint, lemon balm, anise, or fennel oils to the chest rub.

- Precautions: Do not take eucalyptus oil internally.

Ear, Eyes, Mouth & Throat

Modern medicine tends to separate light, hearing, and voice from the rest of the body. Still, the eyes, ears, and mouth condition may reveal information about an individual's overall health. Problems with these organs that persist may indicate the presence of other underlying systemic disorders. For instance, even the orthodox are now acknowledging that glue ear (secretory otitis media) in children is often linked to milk allergies, and all cold sore sufferers are well aware that the Herpes simplex virus flares up when they are exhausted, depressed, or on the verge of catching a cold. According to Chinese theory, hearing symptoms and tinnitus can indicate kidney failure, and chronic mouth complaints or swollen lips can indicate excessive heat in the spleen. While symptomatic treatments may help, addressing the root condition is equally essential. Eye baths of rosewater or weak infusions of eyebright, pot marigold, cornflowers, or strawberry leaves, for example, can benefit tired, strained eyes. Boost illumination conditions, take regular brief breaks from VDU panels or try liver-cleansing herbs as a longer-term alternative.

Similarly, one stye can be treated with marigold compresses or soaking in marigold infusion. Still, if the infection is chronic and ongoing, antimicrobial remedies or toxin-fighting herbs such as burdock, cleavers, echinacea, or garlic may be needed. Similarly, mouth ulcers may be the product of local injury and infection. They can be treated with herbs such as purple sage and myrrh. Still, chronic ulcers can indicate a weakened immune system or underlying yeast infections (candidiasis), including dietary changes or stimulant herbs.

Earache

It may be linked to a catarrhal disease or an illness. Note: Severe illnesses may lead to deafness, so if symptoms continue, seek competent medical attention.

Key Symptoms

- Pain in one or both ears can be severe.

- Blocked sensation in the ears.
- Buzzing or ringing sounds.
- Excessive waxy discharge.
- Fever.
- Vertigo, nausea if the inner ear is affected.

Remedies

1. Verbascum thapsus—**MULLEIN**

Flowers

- Action: Demulcent and mildly sedative wound herb.
- How to use: Cold infused oil of the flowers can be used as ear drops.
- Combinations: Support with antibiotic herbs like echinacea and anti-catarrhals such as elderflower or goldenseal taken internally.
- Precautions: Do not put anything in the ear if there is a risk that the eardrum has perforated.

2. Pulsatilla vulgaris—**PASQUE FLOWER**

Aerial Parts

- Action: Sedative and analgesic; directionally acting on ears and reproductive system.
- How to use: Take 1–2 ml tincture three times daily.
- Combinations: Combine with anti-catarrhals such as goldenseal or eyebright tinctures.

3. Hydrastis canadensis—**GOLDENSEAL**

Rhizome

- Action: Powerful cooling astringent and anti-catarrhal.
- How to use: Use two 200 mg powder in capsules three times daily or 20 drops of tincture per dose.
- Combinations: Add eyebright powder to capsules.
- Precautions: Avoid pregnancy and high blood pressure; do not exceed the stated dose.

4. Plantago lanceolata—**RIBWORT PLANTAIN**

Leaves

- Action: Tonifies mucous membranes and controls catarrh. Useful for catarrhal conditions of the middle ear.
- How to use: Standard infusion or tincture.
- Combinations: Combine with elderflower tincture and add 10 drops of pasque flower tincture to enhance focus on the ears.

Conjunctivitis & Blepharitis

Blepharitis is an inflammation of the eyelids, whereas conjunctivitis is an inflammation of the conjunctiva (the membrane between the eyeball and lid). Infection, asthma, or physical/chemical irritants may all affect these symptoms.

Key Symptoms

- Gritty feeling in the eye.
- Increased light sensitivity.
- Pain, soreness, and swelling.
- Obvious red or pink eye.

- Discharge that may be watery or contain pus if there is an infection.

Remedies

1. Euphrasia Officinalis—**EYEBRIGHT**

Aerial Parts

- Actions: Astringent, anti-catarrhal, and anti-inflammatory.
- How to use: Use a compress soaked in standard infusion for eyes or 5–10 drops of tincture in an eye bath of boiled and cooled water.
- Combinations: Support with internal antibacterials, such as echinacea, if there is infection.

2. Agrimonia eupatoria—**AGRIMONY**

Aerial Parts

- Actions: Astringent and healing for mucosa; also a liver tonic, which may help the eyes.

- How to use: Use weak infusion (10 g to 500 ml of water) well-strained as an eye bath.
- Combinations: Support with internal antibacterials, such as echinacea, if there is infection.

3. Calendula officinalis—**POT MARIGOLD**

Flower Petals

- Actions: Anti-inflammatory, astringent, wound herb, antiseptic. Helpful for local irritation.
- How to use: Use a compress soaked in a well-diluted tincture; also for bathing styes (5 ml to 50 ml water).

4. Dendranthema x grandiflorum—JU HUA **FLOWERS**

- Actions: Antibacterial, anti-inflammatory, and liver herb. Good for persistent eye problems.
- How to use: Standard infusion or tincture internally.
- Combinations: Combine with eyebright, elderflower, agrimony, self-heal to reduce inflammation and support the liver.

Mouth Ulcers (Aphthous Stomatitis)

White ulcers on the lips, tongue, or gums are frequently caused by a bacterial or fungal infection. They may be linked to an unhealthy intake of sugar or other foods that promote fungal growth. A vitamin deficiency may be shown by broken or cracked lips.

Key Symptoms

- An ulcer is obvious on visual inspection.
- It can be very painful and persistent.

Remedies

1. Commiphora molmol—**MYRRH**

Resin

- Actions: Antimicrobial, astringent, wound herb.
- How to use: 5–10 drops of oil or 5 ml tincture in a glass of warm water as a mouthwash.

- Combinations: Add 5 ml sage or rosemary tincture to the mouthwash or chew bilberries afterward to help disguise the flavor.
- Precautions: Avoid high doses internally in pregnancy.

2. Salvia officinalis Purpurescens Group or Salvia officinalis—**PURPLE or GREEN SAGE**

Leaves

- Actions: Antiseptic and astringent; also suitable for gingivitis and other mouth/gum disorders.
- How to use: Standard infusion as mouthwash or 10 ml tincture in a glass of water.
- Combinations: Add self-heal, echinacea, or rosemary tincture to mouthwash.
- Precautions: Avoid high doses internally in pregnancy.

3. Polygonum bistorta—**BISTORT**

Root

- Actions: Astringent, demulcent, and anti-inflammatory; also for other mouth inflammations.
- How to use: Standard decoction or 5 ml tincture to a glass of water as a mouthwash.
- Combinations: Add self-heal, rosemary, bilberry, wild indigo to mouthwash. For persistent problems, take echinacea or garlic internally (see Infections).

Cold Sores

A small collection of blisters usually on the mouth or face due to the Herpes simplex virus. Once infected with the virus, sores may recur when the system is weakened by infection, stress, or fatigue.

Key Symptoms

- Painful with a characteristic appearance.

Remedies

1. Melaleuca alternifolia—**TEA TREE**

Essential Oil

- Actions: Antibiotic and immune stimulant.
- How to use: Use 10 drops of essential oil in 5 ml of carrier oil and dab onto the affected area as soon as the "tingle" of developing sore starts.
- Combinations: Use as a simple. If sore are recurrent, use immune stimulants, such as Huang qi or Siberian ginseng, to improve stress tolerance. If the sore heralds a cold, take echinacea or garlic internally.
- Precautions: Do not take essential oils internally without professional advice. May cause allergic dermatitis in some people; if in doubt, do a skin test before using medicinally.

2. Lavandula officinalis—**LAVENDER**

Essential Oil

- Actions: Topically antiseptic How to use: use a drop of neat oil directly to the affected area as soon as the "tingle" of developing sore starts.

- Combinations: Use as a simple. If sore are recurrent, use immune stimulants, such as Huang qi or Siberian ginseng, to improve stress tolerance. If the sore heralds a cold, take echinacea or garlic internally.
- Precautions: Do not take essential oils internally without professional advice.

Sore Throats

Pain at the back of the mouth associated with infection or chemical irritants; may be linked with tonsillitis, pharyngitis, or laryngitis.

Key Symptoms

- Pain.
- Difficulty in swallowing.
- Voice may be affected – hoarse or croaking.
- Related fever or cold may be present or starting.
- Inflammation is apparent on inspection.

Remedies

1. Agrimonia eupatoria—**AGRIMONY**

Aerial Parts

- Action: Astringent and healing for the mucosa.
- How to use: Standard infusion as a gargle or use 10 ml tincture in a glass of warm water.
- Combinations: Add 5 ml of echinacea, purple sage, or rosemary tincture to the gargle.

2. Alchemilla Vulgaris—**LADY'S MANTLE**

Leaves

- Action: Astringent and reduces inflammation; helpful for laryngitis.
- How to use: Standard infusion as a gargle or use 10 ml tincture in a glass of warm water.
- Combinations: Add 5 ml of rosemary or purple sage tincture or no more than 5 drops of cayenne tincture to the gargle.

- Precautions: Avoid large internal doses in pregnancy.

3. Echinacea spp.—**ECHINACEA**

Root or Leaves

- Action: Antibacterial and astringent; useful for all throat problems, including tonsillitis.
- How to use: Use 5 ml of tincture in a glass of warm water as a gargle. Swallow the gargle to help combat infection.

4. Terminalia belerica—**BIBHITAKI**

Fruit

- Actions: Closely associated in Ayurvedic tradition with both the throat and voice, bibhitaki fruits are astringent, antiseptic, and cooling.
- How to use: Take 1 teaspoon of powder in honey for sore throats and vocal problems; use the infusion or juice as a gargle Combinations: Use as a simple or add antimicrobials such as 5 ml of echinacea infusion to the gargle to combat infection.
- Precautions: Avoid pregnancy and severe exhaustion.

Tonsillitis

Tonsil inflammation is normally caused by a bacterial or viral infection. Quinsy (peritonsillar abscess) will exacerbate things, necessitating a surgical incision to drain the fluid.

Key Symptoms

- Sore throat.
- Difficulty swallowing.
- Fever.
- Tonsils may be enlarged or suppurating on inspection.

Remedies

1. Galium aparine—**CLEAVERS**

Aerial Parts

- Action: Lymphatic cleanser and alterative; useful lymphatic problems including glandular fever and adenoids.

- How to use: Use 10 ml of fresh juice three times daily or standard infusion internally.
- Combinations: Add additional antibacterial tinctures such as 10 drops of goldenseal or poke root, or up to 10 ml of echinacea to the juice internally; use gargles as suggested for "sore throat" above.

2. Phytolacca Americana—**POKE ROOT**

Dried Root

- Action: Anti-catarrhal and cleansing for the lymphatic system; reduces lymphatic swellings.
- How to use: 10–20 drops of tincture made from the dried root, three times daily.
- Combinations: Use 10 ml of cleaver juice or add additional antibacterial tinctures such as 10 ml echinacea.
- Precautions: Large doses are emetic and purgative – do not exceed the stated dose. Do not use any part of the fresh plant, which is toxic.

3. Baptisia tinctorial—**WILD INDIGO**

Leaves and Root

- Action: Antimicrobial, anti-catarrhal, cleansing for lymphatics; good for persistent infection.
- How to use: 10–20 drops of a tincture, three times daily taken internally.
- Combinations: Combine with cleaver juice of echinacea tincture to enhance action.
- Precautions: Large doses can cause nausea—do not exceed the stated dose.

4. Gnaphalium uliginosum—**MARSH CUDWEED**

Leaves

- Action: Anti-inflammatory and tonifying for the mucosa; also for laryngitis, pharyngitis, and quinsy.
- How to use: Take a standard infusion or tincture internally and use it as a gargle.
- Combinations: Combine with cleaver juice of echinacea tincture to enhance action.

Skin & Hair

Although medical medicine also uses hydrocortisone creams to treat skin issues, a herbal treatment relies on maintaining internal equilibrium, often with washing or cooling herbs, rather than using external treatments that can temporarily relieve symptoms but do little to address the underlying cause of the issue. Ayurvedic medicine recognizes the same need for rebalancing: too much pitta (fire) causes the blood to overheat and poison the skin; too much Vata (wind) causes dryness and itching, and too much Kapha (damp) causes vomiting or oozing sores. Herbs that are calming, drying, or moistening, and a proper diet, are used to treat the condition. Dry, flaking eczema, for example, will be handled with herbs to cool and raise body fluids, while the Chinese equate skin with the lung, wei qi (defense energy), and body fluids. This technique has shown promising results in trials at a London hospital. Skin infections caused by fungi or parasites are considered a weakness of the wei qi and are treated with immunostimulants and antimicrobials. For chronic fungal infections, Western herbalism adopts a similar approach, implying some structural deficiency that can be handled with tonic herbs and immunostimulants rather than the use of symptomatic antifungals. Hair issues may also be a symptom of other physical flaws. Hair is associated with the kidneys in Chinese medicine, so premature graying of the hair is associated with decreased kidney energy and should be handled with tonics rather than colorants.

Eczema

Allergies, nervous stress, and chemical/metal irritants may all cause skin inflammation. If a local irritant (such as a metal watch strap) is present, it can be very localized, but allergic eczema can affect any part of the body. Body crevices, such as the folds of the elbows or under the breasts, are often affected.

Key Symptoms

- Red, inflamed patches on the skin.
- It can be itchy.
- May start oozing serum from the raw surface.
- Crusts of serum can be formed.
- Lesions may bleed in acute conditions.

Remedies

1. Stellaria media—**CHICKWEED**

Aerial Parts

- Actions: Soothing and slightly astringent wound herb to ease irritation and help heal lesions.
- How to use: Apply ointment or cream as required; add infused oil to the bathwater.
- Combinations: Use externally as a simple.

2. Oenothera biennis—**EVENING PRIMROSE**

Seed Oil

- Actions: Contains essential fatty acids that are needed to maintain healthy tissues.
- How to use: In capsules: 1–2 g daily for children; 3 g for adults.
- Combinations: Use as a simple.

3. Paeonia lactiflora—RED PEONY (Chi Shao Yao)

Root

- Actions: Cools and stimulates blood flow; useful for "hot" conditions.
- How to use: Standard decoction or tincture: best combined with other herbs.
- Combinations: Combine with additional cooling remedies such as sheng di huang, heartsease, mu dan pi, fang feng, and mu tong.

4. Arctium lappa—**BURDOCK**

Leaf

- Actions: Cleansing, diuretic, and laxative. Good for any toxic skin condition, especially dry, scaling eczema.
- How to use: Standard decoction of the root or up to 4 ml of the tincture three times daily.
- Combinations: Combine with other cleansing remedies such as yellow dock, figwort cleavers, heartsease, and red clover tinctures.

5. Urtica dioica—**STINGING NETTLE**

Aerial Parts

- Actions: Astringent, tonic, and circulatory stimulant; useful if eczema is associated with poor circulation.
- How to use: Standard infusion or tincture. Also, like cream or ointment.
- Combinations: Use a simple combination with other cleansing herbs such as heartsease, red clover, figwort, and cleavers tinctures.

Acne

Inflammation of the sebaceous glands in the skin may begin with blackheads, most frequent in adolescents.

Key Symptoms

- Inflamed pustules.
- Often excessive oiliness of the skin.
- In severe cases, there may be infected cysts and scarring.

Remedies

1. Allium sativa—**GARLIC**

Clove

- Actions: Antibacterial and antifungal; good antiseptic action for infected skin conditions How to use: Rub the affected area directly with a cut clove.
- Combinations: Use as a simple; eat parsley to limit garlic odor – and use garlic in cooking.
- Precautions: Because of the odor, this is best done at night.

2. Melaleuca alternifolia—**TEA TREE**

Essential Oil

- Actions: Potent antibacterial for infected skin conditions.
- How to use: Use 10 ml of tea tree oil in 100 ml of water or a 50:50 mixture of rosewater and distilled witch-hazel as a lotion.
- Combinations: Use as a simple and take tinctures of cleavers, yellow dock, burdock, or echinacea internally.

- Precautions: Do not take essential oils internally without professional advice.
- May cause allergic dermatitis in some people; if in doubt, do a skin test before using medicinally.

3. Brassica oleracea —**CABBAGE**

Leaf

- Actions: Antibacterial and anti-inflammatory; nutritive and healing.
- How to use: Mix 250 g of fresh leaves and 250 ml of distilled witch hazel in a blender; strain and add 2 drops of lemon oil and use as a lotion.
- Combinations: Use as a simple and take tinctures of cleavers, yellow dock, burdock, or echinacea internally.

Verrucas and Warts

Growth in the outer layer of the skin due to a virus.

Key Symptoms

- Obvious growth.
- Can spread by contact.
- It may be persistent.

Remedies

1. Thuja occidentalis—**ARBOR VITAE**

Leaf Tips

- Actions: Volatile oil contains thujone, which is strongly antiseptic and effective against many topical fungal and viral infections.
- How to use: Use drops of the tincture neat on verrucas or warts; it can also be made into an ointment. Repeat often.
- Precautions: Avoid pregnancy.

2. Chelidonium majus—**GREATER CELANDINE**

Sap

- Actions: Potent antiviral to destroy warts.
- How to use: Squeeze the fresh sap from the stems directly to the wart; repeat at least twice a day, and even longstanding warts will generally clear in 2–3 weeks.
- Combinations: Use as a simple; dandelion stem sap can be used similarly.
- Precautions: Do not take it internally or use any part of the plant in pregnancy; avoid touching surrounding skin with too much sap.

Psoriasis

It is caused by an overabundance of skin keratinocytes that do not develop into natural keratin; it is linked to immune deficiency and may happen after a streptococcal infection or a skin injury. It is often attributed to a tense, lonely personality that does not want to get attached to other people, and it is exacerbated by tension and concern. Psoriasis is a disease that also runs through families.

Key Symptoms

- Red skin patches often with silver-colored scales.
- The cycle of remission and reoccurrence.

Remedies

1. Galium aparine—**CLEAVERS**

Aerial Parts

- Actions: Cleansing, diuretic, and astringent useful for many types of skin problems.
- How to use: Use 10 ml fresh juice three times daily or standard infusion. Also externally as ointment or cream.
- Combinations: Combine well with red clover to help overproduce cells and cleansing stimulants such as figwort or stinging nettles in the infusion.

2. Iris versicolor—**BLUE FLAG**

Rhizome

- Actions: Anti-inflammatory and cleansing of both blood and lymphatic systems; a favorite with the physiomedicalists and stimulating liver.
- How to use: Use in decoction (half a teaspoon per cup in half cup doses) or tincture.
- Combinations: With cleansing remedies such as poke root and yellow dock, add valerian to the decoction. If stress or anxiety are significant factors, use aloe vera sap or slippery elm powder as a topical treatment.

3. Scrophularia nodosa—**FIGWORT**

Aerial Parts

- Actions: Anti-inflammatory, cleansing, and circulatory stimulant: good for many chronic skin conditions.
- How to use: Standard infusion or tincture.
- Combinations: Use red clover or heartsease to help normalize skin growth or cleansing herbs such as cleavers and yellow dock.

- Precautions: Avoid certain heart conditions such as tachycardia.

4. Trifolium pratense—**RED CLOVER**

Flowers

- Actions: Cleansing and diuretic useful for many skin problems, including eczema.
- How to use: Standard infusion or tincture also externally in creams and ointments
- Combinations: Combine with cleavers in infusion or add 2 ml yellow dock or 10 drops arborvitae to tinctures.

5. Rumex Crispus—**YELLOW DOCK**

Root

- Actions: Cleansing diuretic and laxative; stimulates bile flow and clears toxins.
- How to use: Standard decoction or tincture.
- Combinations: Combine with burdock and figwort tinctures.
- Precautions: Avoid high doses in pregnancy.

Fungal Infections

Microorganisms including Microsporum, Trichophyton, and Epidermophyton spp. Cause ringworm, athlete's foot, and other fungal infections. They can affect any part of the body, but the toes, nails, and scalp are the most often affected.

Key Symptoms

- Very irritant.
- Red patches.
- The skin may be scaly and peeling.

Remedies

1. Calendula officinalis—**POT MARIGOLD**

Flower Petals

- Action: Antifungal and astringent; wound herb and soothing for dry or inflamed skin.

- How to use: Use as cream or ointment or a standard infusion in a footbath or as a wash.
- Combination: Add 5 ml of tea tree oil to 500 ml of pot marigold infusion used as a wash.

Commiphora molmol—MYRRH

Resin or Essential Oil

- Action: Antifungal, immune stimulant, and astringent How to use: Use 10 drops of oil or 10 ml tincture to 100 ml water as a wash. Take up to 20 drops of tincture in water three times daily.
- Combination: Pot marigold, echinacea, arborvitae tincture three times daily internally Precautions: Do not take essential oils internally. Avoid internally in pregnancy.

2. Aloe vera—**ALOE VERA**

Gel

- Action: Demulcent, cooling for irritated skin, antiparasitic, also for infestations such as scabies.
- How to use: Use the sap from a fresh leaf directly on the affected area; aloe gel is available commercially.

Hair Loss – Alopecia

Alopecia can be total or localized to particular patches; mild hair loss problems can be linked to vitamin deficiency.

Key Symptoms

- Excessive loose hairs; a small loss is quite normal.
- Bald patches.

Remedies

1. Arnica montana—**ARNICA**

Flowers

- Actions: Stimulates blood circulation.

- How to use: Use as cream or ointment on affected areas of the scalp, or use 5 ml of 1:10 tincture in 500 ml warm water as a rinse.
- Combination: Support with nerves (see p. 200) taken internally to combat stress and Vitamin B supplements. Drink cleansing infusions of burdock, stinging nettle, cleavers, or red clover.
- Precautions: Do not use it on broken skin or take it internally.

2. Artemisia abrotanum—**SOUTHERNWOOD**

Aerial Parts

- Action: Traditional remedy to stimulate hair growth – although there is no scientific basis for this action.
- How to use: Take 10–20 drops of tincture internally three times daily; use a standard infusion as a hair rinse.
- Combination: Add stinging nettles, rosemary, or sage infusions to the hair rinse; take mineral supplements and vitamin B.
- Precautions: Avoid completely in pregnancy or if trying to conceive.

Premature Graying

It can be an inherited tendency or associated with stress or premature menopause.

Key Symptoms

• Hair starts to lose its color in the twenties or thirties.

Remedies

1. Salvia officinalis Purpurescens group or Salvia officinalis — **PURPLE or GREEN SAGE**

Leaves

- Action: Traditionally used to restore color – possibly associated with general tonic and hormonal properties of sage.
- How to use: Standard infusion internally and as a hair rinse.
- Combination: Add rosemary and stinging nettles to the infusion or rinse.
- Precautions: Avoid high doses internally in pregnancy.

2. Polygonum multiflorum—**HE SHOU WU**

Root

- Action: Kidney tonic used in China for premature menopause early graying hair.
- How to use: Standard decoction or tincture taken internally (up to 15 ml daily).
- Combination: Can be used as a simple or combined with Nu Zhen Zi, shu di huang, and licorice tinctures.
- Precautions: Avoid if also suffering from diarrhea.

Dandruff

Small flakes of dead skin on the scalp; may be associated with seborrheic dermatitis and underlying yeast infections.

Key Symptoms

- Obvious scurf on collars and combs.

- Hair may be dry and brittle or greasy with yellow dandruff flakes.

Remedies

1. Rosmarinus officinalis—**ROSEMARY**

Aerial Parts

- Action: Astringent, antiseptic, and circulatory stimulant; also useful for psoriasis affecting the scalp.
- How to use: Standard infusion as a hair rinse; or macerate 15 g rosemary in 250 ml shampoo for 2 weeks; strain before using.
- Combination: Add stinging nettle root to infusion for hair rinse.

2. Quillaja saponaria—**SOAP BARK**

Bark

- Actions: Rich in saponins – cleansing and anti-inflammatory.

- How to use: Mix 500 ml of standard decoction with 200 g of soft soap to use as shampoo.
- Precautions: Large internal doses can cause digestive tract irritation and inflammations.

Heart, Blood & Circulation

The heart was viewed as something more than just an effective pump for controlling blood supply in ancient medical practices. It is the seat of the mind, the dwelling of atman – the eternal self or essence of eternal life – in Ayurvedic medicine, and it stores shén: the spirit and sense of consciousness in Chinese medicine. Disharmonies of shén are blamed in Chinese medicine for what modern Western medicine may consider as a mental disease or nervous disorders, and herbs like fu ling, which is used as a sedative to "pacify the heart" in insomnia and palpitations, may be recommended.

Western heart herbs have a more traditional range of actions: scientists have been researching herbal heart remedies since William Withering discovered foxglove (Digitalis purpurea) as a potent heart cure in 1768. Others are highly powerful and essential in medical medicine, while some are safe to use at home, such as hawthorn and linden flower tea, which can treat high blood pressure in pregnant women.

Vasodilators, which soften and expand blood flow; diuretics, which decrease blood flow; and cardiac depressants, which slow the heart rate, are both herbal treatments for hypertension. Hypertension, according to Chinese medicine, is linked to prolonged liver fire flaring, for example. Herbs may also help regulate cholesterol levels, with many lowering abnormally elevated serum lipid levels and preventing atherosclerosis – but a healthier diet, active lifestyle, and pollution-free atmosphere will possibly avoid this from becoming an issue for most people.

High Blood Pressure

Hypertension can be seen as a symptom of a larger body imbalance rather than a particular illness. It may be linked to other underlying conditions like atherosclerosis, heart disease, or liver issues.

Key Symptoms

- Headaches.
- Eye problems.
- Dizziness or fainting spells.
- Raised blood pressure reading on repeated examination.
- Diastolic (lower reading) greater than 90–95 mm Hg.

Note: Do not replace orthodox medication with herbs without consulting your practitioner.

Remedies

1. Viburnum opulus—**GUELDER ROSE**

Bark

- Action: Smooth muscle relaxant for the vascular system; lowers the diastolic pressure.
- How to use: Standard decoction or tincture.

- Combinations: Combines with linden flowers if there is atherosclerosis, or valerian or passionflower is stress is involved; add hawthorn as a heart tonic if required.

2. Stachys officinalis—**WOOD BETONY**

Aerial Parts

- Action: Circulatory tonic, relaxant, and sedative; calms the heart.
- How to use: Standard infusion or tincture.
- Combinations: Combines with linden flowers if there is atherosclerosis or with guelder rose to relax blood vessels; add valerian or passionflower if stress is involved.
- Precautions: Uterine stimulant, so avoid high doses in pregnancy.

3. Dendranthema x grandiflorum—**JU HUA**

Flowers

- Action: Dilates the coronary artery and increases blood flow; also clears liver heat which can cause hypertension.

- How to use: Standard infusion or tincture.
- Combinations: Combine with liver herbs such as gou qi zi and diuretics like a dandelion leaf and fu ling.

4. Crataegus spp.—**HAWTHORN**

Berries or Flowering Tops

- Action: Improves coronary circulation and strengthens heart muscles; useful tincture for angina pectoris. Helps stabilize BP as cardiac function improves.
- How to use: Standard infusion or tincture.
- Combinations: Combines well in teas with linden flowers and yarrow, or with guelder rose to relax blood vessels; add valerian or passionflower if stress is involved.

1. Tilia x Europaea—**LINDEN**

Flowers

- Action: Peripheral vasodilator with a healing effect on blood vessels; reputed prophylactic against arteriosclerosis.

- How to use: Standard infusion or up to 10 ml tincture daily.
- Combinations: Combine with hawthorn as a cardiac tonic or with ginkgo and linden flowers if arteriosclerosis is significant.

Low Blood Pressure

Often not considered serious by doctors, but hypotension can be a significant health problem.

Key Symptoms

- General tiredness.
- Weak constitution.
- Dizziness and/or fainting spells.
- Palpitations and cardiac arrhythmias.
- It can be serious if the systolic (upper) reading is consistently below 110 mm Hg, seeking professional help.

Remedies

2. Cytisus scoparius—**BROOM**

Flowering Tops

- Action: Regulates heartbeat steadying the arrhythmias that can be associated with low BP and heart failure.
- How to use: Use 15 g to 500 ml water for infusions or up to 5 ml tincture daily.
- Combinations: Use tonics such as hawthorn.
- Precautions: Avoid pregnancy.

3. Convallaria majalis—**LILY-OF-THE-VALLEY**

Leaves

- Action: Stimulates heart contractions and improves efficiency; useful for weak, failing, and elderly hearts.
- How to use: Restricted to professional use in some geographies. The maximum dose in the UK is 20 drops of a 1:5 tincture three times daily.
- Combinations are always combined with a diuretic such as dandelion leaf; heart tonics such as hawthorn are often added.

- Precautions: High doses are emetic and purgative; take only as prescribed.

4. Leonurus cardiac—**MOTHERWORT**

Leaves

- Action: Relaxing for palpitations and arrhythmias; also has a stimulating action on the heart.
- How to use: Standard infusion or tincture.
- Combinations: Combine with rosemary as a tonic or add sedatives such as passionflower for stress-related problems.
- Precautions: Avoid pregnancy.

Varicose Veins

Leg veins that are swollen or extended are linked to low venous return or high abdominal pressure (obesity and pregnancy).

Key Symptoms

- Obvious enlarged and stretched veins.
- Pain in the legs.

Remedies

1. Melilotus officinale—**KING'S CLOVER**

Aerial Parts

- Actions: A good venous tonic, rich in coumarin-like compounds; anti-coagulant and anti-inflammatory.
- How to use: Use a standard infusion; up to 3 ml of tincture three times a day; externally as cream; or use 10% tincture in witch-hazel or rosewater.
- Combinations: Use liver herbs (like goldenseal) if sluggish digestion is a contributing factor; add pot marigold to creams and compresses.

- Precautions: Do not use warfarin or similar anti-coagulant drugs to thin the blood or any problem with the blood's ability to clot.

2. Aesculus hippocastanum—**HORSE CHESTNUT**

Seed

- Action: Astringent and internally strengthening to the blood vessels, possibly due to the presence of medicine.
- How to use: Take up to 2.5 ml of tincture three times a day; use dilute tincture for compresses.
- Combinations: Use liver herbs (like goldenseal) if sluggish digestion is a contributing factor; add distilled witch-hazel to compresses.
- Precautions: Seed coatings of horse chestnut can be toxic; peel before use if using large quantities.

Poor Circulation

It may be a sign of a more serious heart disorder but is often simply an inherited tendency and not a major problem.

Key Symptoms

- Exceptionally cold hands and feet.
- The tendency for chilblains.
- Raynaud's phenomenon ("dead" or white fingers).

Remedies

1. Zanthoxylum americanum—**PRICKLY ASH**

Bark

- Action: Diaphoretic and circulatory stimulant; warming for all cold conditions.
- How to use: Use 15 g to 600 ml water for decoctions; take up to 5 ml tincture daily.
- Combinations: Add angelica root or a pinch of cinnamon powder to decoctions, or combine with rosemary tincture.

2. Cinnamonum cassia—**GUI ZHI**

Twigs

- Action: Warming, diaphoretic; encourages both blood and qi circulation.
- How to use: Standard decoction or tincture.
- Combinations: Combines well with ginger in decoction or add rosemary or ginkgo to tinctures.
- Precautions: Avoid high doses in pregnancy.

3. Capsicum frutescens—**CAYENNE**

Fruit

- Action: Heating, diaphoretic, and a strong circulatory stimulant.
- How to use: Use 30–50 mg to 500 ml of water for infusions; up to 1 ml of a 1:20 tincture three times daily; externally as infused oil in massage.
- Combinations: Combine with other warming stimulants such as angelica root or bayberry decoctions.
- Precautions: Do not exceed the stated dose.

4. Zingiber officinale—**GINGER**

Root

- Action: Strong circulatory stimulant, diaphoretic, and vasodilator; very warming.
- How to use: Use up to 10 g fresh root to 600 ml water for decoctions and footbaths; up to 2 ml of a 1:20 tincture three times daily.
- Combinations: Add rosemary or gui Zhi to decoctions or take a circulatory stimulant such as ginkgo.

Palpitations & Angina Pectoris

Palpitations are merely a feeling of being conscious of one's pulse, which may be triggered by shock, exercise, alcohol, or excitement. Angina pectoris is caused by a narrowing of the coronary artery, which restricts blood flow to the heart; palpitations can signal the start of an attack.

Key Symptoms

- Angina attacks usually involve a heavy, pressing pain in the chest which may radiate to the jaw or left arm.
- Breathlessness, panic.

Important: Angina pectoris always requires professional treatment.

Remedies

1. Alpinia galangal—**GALANGAL**

Root

- Actions: Traditional heart remedy, now known to ease heart pains, dizziness, and fatigue and reduce the symptoms of angina pectoris.
- How to use: Take in tablets, tinctures, or decoctions; a few drops of neat tincture on the tongue may help avert an angina attack.
- Combinations: Use hawthorn berries, khella, and prickly ash in decoctions and tinctures.

2. Leonurus cardiac—**MOTHERWORT**

Aerial Parts

- Actions: Heart tonic and relaxant to combat feelings of panic and normalize heartbeat in palpitations.
- How to use: Take in tinctures or infusions.
- Combinations: Use hawthorn flowers and linden in infusions; add rose petals or skullcap for feelings of panic or shock causing palpitations.
- Precautions: Avoid pregnancy.

3. Passiflora incarnate—**PASSION FLOWER**

Aerial Parts

- Actions: Sedative and calming, heart tonic, and relaxant for blood vessels.
- How to use: Take in infusions, tablets, and tinctures.
- Combinations: Use hawthorn and linden as an infusion for everyday drinking in angina pectoris; add skullcap or wood

betony for palpitations associated with shock or emotional upsets.

- Precautions: Use only low doses in pregnancy; may cause drowsiness.

Iron Deficient Anemia

Low hemoglobin levels can be due to poor diet, hemorrhage (or heavy menstrual bleeding), or digestive disorders.

Key Symptoms

- Breathlessness.
- Very pale fingernails and inner eyelids.
- Rheumatic-type pains.
- Palpitations.

Remedies

1. Urtica dioica—**STINGING NETTLES**

Aerial Parts

- Actions: Rich in iron, other minerals, and vitamins; highly nutritious.
- How to use: 10 ml of juice three times daily; use a standard infusion or make nettle soup.
- Combinations: Use as a simple but add other iron-rich foods to the diet, such as liver, parsley, watercress, or apricots. Supplements of ashwagandha can also help.

2. Angelica polypharmacy var. Sinensis—**DANG GUI**

Root

- Actions: Nourishes the blood and invigorates the circulation; contains vitamin B12 and folic acid, which can also help pernicious anemia.
- How to use: Standard decoction and tincture.
- Combinations: Can combine with shu di huang and he shou wu. Add other iron-rich foods to the diet, such as liver, parsley, watercress, or apricots. Supplements of ashwagandha can also help.
- Precautions: Avoid pregnancy.

High Cholesterol

Excessive blood lipid levels (such as cholesterol) may contribute to atherosclerosis and an elevated likelihood of heart disease. Excess saturated fat in the diet is also linked to this condition; the family history is crucial. Cholesterol is needed for a variety of body transport mechanisms and is not dangerous in and of itself. If dietary cholesterol is insufficient, the body can produce enough to maintain equilibrium.

Key Symptoms

• Generally only diagnosed after blood tests.

Remedies

1. Camellia sinensis —**GREEN or OOLONG TEA**

Leaf

- Actions: Phenols inhibit cholesterol absorption; circulatory stimulant and tonic for blood vessels helping to prevent atherosclerosis.

- How to use: 1–2 teaspoons per cup of boiling water as an infusion.
- Combinations: Use as a simple. Pu Erh is the most effective variety of oolong tea for reducing cholesterol levels.
- Precautions: Limit to 2 cups daily in hypertension and pregnancy.

2. Allium sativa—**GARLIC**

Clove

- Actions: Reduces serum cholesterol levels and has been shown to help prevent repeat heart attacks and atherosclerosis.
- How to use: 1 clove daily; 2 g powdered garlic in capsules if there is a high risk of heart attacks.
- Combinations: Use as a simple or in cooking. Limit intake of high cholesterol foods and saturated fats.

3. Avena sativa—**OATS**

Seed

- Actions: Effectively reduces serum cholesterol levels, particularly low-density lipoproteins.
- How to use: Make oatmeal porridge or add 25 g of oat bran to breakfast cereal.
- Combinations: Use as a simple. Limit intake of high cholesterol foods and saturated fats.

Capillary Fragility

Weakness in the blood vessel walls.

Key Symptoms

- Tendency to bruise easily.
- Retinal hemorrhages.
- Petechiae (flat dark red spots caused by bleeding into the skin).

Remedies

1. Fagopyrum esculentum—**BUCKWHEAT**

Seed

- Action: Rich in rutin, which tonifies and repairs the arteriole walls; specific for retinal hemorrhage.
- How to use: Standard infusion or tincture; commercial tablets also available.
- Combinations: Use 10 ml of horsetail juice per dose.

2. Viola tricolor—**HEARTSEASE**

Aerial Parts

- Actions: Contains flavonoids, which strengthen the capillary walls.
- How to use: Standard infusion or tincture.
- Combinations: Use 10 ml of horsetail juice per dose or add yarrow or ribwort plantain to infusions.

Digestive Problems

Good digestion is essential for good health; it deprives the body of essential nutrients and causes toxic excretion products to build up. According to Ayurvedic philosophy, these excretion products cause the three humors – pitta, Vata, and Kapha – which may account for most disease states if they are out of control. According to Ayurvedic philosophy, well-being depends on the Agni, or digestive fire, staying solid and vigorous. The liver is identified with the skin, vision, energy circulation, blood flow, tendons, nails, menstrual diseases, and mental function in Chinese five element theory (see pp. 5–8). At the same time, the spleen and stomach are associated with not only digestion but also blood vessels, nerves, tongue, memory, and purpose. As a result, digestive system imbalances can be linked to various seemingly unrelated physical and emotional effects. In the West, too, herbal medicine has long focused on digestive function, echoing, perhaps, the medieval maxim that "death dwells in the bowels." Herbs will include a remarkable variety of tonics, stimulants, carminatives, and relaxants to maintain good work. Bitter remedies like gentian or barberry promote digestion, while liver tonics like milk thistle can help restore damage by stimulating cell formation. Strong purgatives used in traditional medicine, such as senna and cascara, are often herbal, but gentler laxatives are preferred.

The nervous system, which stimulates acid or enzyme formation, peristaltic gut contractions (which carry food and feces along), and blood flow, which collects the absorbed nutrients, all play a role in proper digestion. Many of the more common herbal digestive treatments, such as lemon balm, chamomile, hops, rosemary, guelder rose, vervain, and lavender, work on the nervous system well and can help with stress-related issues, including colitis and hyperacidity.

Note: If you notice a difference in the daily bowel routine that lasts more than two to three days or happens unexpectedly, seek medical advice.

Constipation

Generally a symptom of other health issues, it may be caused by a healthy diet, slow intestinal activity, or low muscle tone, or it may be caused by nervous stress that prevents regular bowel movement.

Key Symptoms

- Lack of bowel motions for more than 24 hours.

- Low abdominal pain or griping.
- Difficulty in passing stool.

Remedies

1. Rheum palmatum—**RHUBARB**

Root

- Actions: Contains anthraquinones, which irritate the gut, increasing peristalsis.
- How to use: 10–15 g to 600 ml water as decoction; 2 ml tincture up to three times a day.
- Combinations: Add 1–2 ml of fennel, lemon balm, or chamomile tincture per dose or decoctions to combat any griping; enhance with mild laxatives such as butternut, yellow dock, or licorice, or add senna pods in more severe cases.
- Precautions: Avoid pregnancy, arthritic conditions, or gout.

2. Viburnum opulus—**GUELDER ROSE**

Bark

- Actions: Smooth muscle relaxant; useful if constipation is linked to visceral tension.
- How to use: Standard decoction or tincture.
- Combinations: Add 1–2 ml of fennel, lemon balm, or chamomile tincture per dose or decoctions to combat any griping; enhance with mild laxatives such as butternut, yellow dock, or licorice, or add senna pods in more severe cases.

3. Plantago psyllium and Plantago ovata—**PSYLLIUM and ISPHAGULA**

Seed

- Actions: Mucilaginous and bulking laxative which lubricates the bowel; useful if the stool is dry.
- How to use: Use 1 teaspoon of seeds in a cup of boiling water; allow to cool and then drink (inc. seeds), repeat once or twice a day.
- Combinations: Use as a simple or mix 2:1 with linseed.

Diarrhea

Sometimes a symptom of other digestive system imbalances, but it may also be triggered by apparent food poisoning or infection. Suspect food is commonly visible in food poisoning, with those who shared the meal being infected as well. However, an illness can quickly be contacted by other members of the family.

Key Symptoms

- Loose and frequent stools.
- Abdominal cramps or griping pains.

Remedies

1. Potentilla erecta—**TORMENTIL**

Root

- Action: Contains up to 20% tannins, making the herb very astringent and reducing the inflammation and irritation associated with diarrhea.

- How to use: 20 g to 600 ml water as decoction; 2–3 ml of tincture up to three times a day.
- Combinations: Add soothing herbs such as ribwort plantain or marshmallow root to ease any gut inflammation.

2. Agrimonia eupatoria—**AGRIMONY**

Aerial Parts

- Action: Stringent and healing for any intestinal tract inflammation, especially suitable for children.
- How to use: Standard infusion or tincture.
- Combinations: Add soothing herbs such as ribwort plantain or marshmallow root to ease any gut inflammation; use bilberry or bistort to increase astringency.

3. Geranium maculatum—**AMERICAN CRANESBILL**

Herb or Root

- Actions: Astringent but gentle enough for children, the elderly, and debilitated.
- How to use: Leaf: standard infusion or tincture.

- Root: 20 g to 600 ml water for decoction; 2–3 ml of tincture three times a day.
- Combinations: Add soothing herbs such as ribwort plantain, meadowsweet, or marshmallow root to ease any inflammation of the gut; use bilberry or bistort to increase astringency.

Gastritis

Inflammation of the gastric mucosa, which, if persistent, can lead to ulceration eventually. It may be due to dietary factors.

Key Symptoms

- Heartburn and acid reflux.
- Persistent vomiting in acute gastritis.
- Diarrhea and abdominal discomfort.

Remedies

1. Althaea Officinalis—**MARSHMALLOW**

Root

- Actions: Soothing and demulcent for irritated mucus membranes; healing for damaged tissue.
- How to use: Use a maceration or tincture made from fresh herbs or powder.
- Combinations: Use meadowsweet with a pinch of cinnamon; combine with carminatives such as fennel and peppermint infusions.

2. Ulmus fulva—**SLIPPERY ELM**

Bark

- Actions: Demulcent to soothe irritated mucosa; also nutritive for debilitating conditions.
- How to use: Up to 5 g of powdered bark in capsules or mixed with water before meals.
- Combinations: Can be combined with an equal amount of powdered marshmallow root.

3. Filipendula ulmaria—**MEADOWSWEET**

Aerial Parts

- Actions: Anti-inflammatory reduces stomach acid secretions and is soothing and healing for the gastric mucosa.
- How to use: Standard infusion, fluid extract or tincture 5 ml tincture daily.
- Combinations: Increase astringency with 10 drops of bistort or American cranesbill tincture or soothe with 10 drops of licorice per dose. Add extra anti-inflammatories, such as pot marigold, if desired.
- Precautions: Avoid in cases of salicylate sensitivity.

Peptic/Duodenal Ulcers

Ulceration of the stomach or duodenal mucous membranes is now associated with the Heliobacter pylori bacterium, associated with stress and dietary abuse.

Key Symptoms

- Easily located pain in the upper abdomen.
- Pain often worse at night or when hungry.

- Possible nausea, heartburn, flatulence, and weight loss.

Remedies

1. Leptospermum scoparium—**NEW ZEALAND TEA TREE** (MANUKA or KAHIKATOA)

Pollen, Flowers, Leaves, or Bark

- Actions: Studies in New Zealand suggest that antimicrobial manuka honey effectively kills the Heliobacter bacterium. How to use: Take 1½ teaspoons of manuka honey twice a day or use the flowers and leaves in infusions or the bark in decoctions.
- Combinations: Add other antibacterials such as echinacea, blue flag, or thyme; add soothing demulcents such as marshmallow root or licorice as decoctions.

2. Glycyrrhiza glabra—**LICORICE**

Root

- Actions: Anti-inflammatory; produces a viscous mucus which coats and protects the stomach wall and limits acid production.
- How to use: Standard decoction, tincture, or fluid extracts; juice sticks can be sucked like sweets.
- Combinations: In severe cases, add extra soothing herbs such as marshmallow root or slippery elm or add anti-inflammatories such as meadowsweet or pot marigold.
- Precautions: Avoid in cases of high blood pressure or if taking digoxin-based drugs.

Inflamed Gallbladder

Cholecystitis may be chronic or acute and is often linked to high-fat consumption.

Key Symptoms

- Constant, severe upper abdominal pain often radiating to the shoulder.
- Sweating, nausea, erratic breathing.

Remedies

1. Berberis vulgaris—**BARBERRY**

Bark

- Actions: Stimulates bile flow and eases liver congestion; bitter and laxative.
- How to use: 15 g of herb to 600 ml water for decoctions or up to 8 ml tincture daily.
- Combinations: Combine with anti-inflammatories such as goldenseal (5 drops of tincture per dose) and add liver tonics such as vervain infusion or globe artichoke juice.
- Precautions: Avoid pregnancy.

2. Chionanthus virginicus—**FRINGE TREE**

Bark

- Actions: Stimulates bile flow and liver function; laxative and cleansing.

- How to use: Use a standard decoction in tablespoon doses or up to 5 ml tincture daily.
- Combinations: Combine with bitters, liver tonics, or stimulants such as dandelion root, milk thistle, chicory, globe artichoke, or centaury, plus anti-inflammatories like pot marigold.

Gallstones

Made of bile pigment and/or cholesterol that become lodged in the bile duct.

Key Symptoms

- Brief attacks of severe upper abdominal pain.
- Most common in the "fair, fat, forty, female, and flatulent."
- Jaundice, indigestion, vomiting.

Remedies

1. Peumus boldo—BOLDO

Leaves

- Actions: Stimulates bile flow and liver activity, reduces inflammation, and helps protect the liver.
- How to use: Use 10–30 drops of tincture per dose or half a teaspoon of dried leaves to two cups of an infusion taken in half-cup doses.
- Combinations: Traditionally combined with barberry and fringe tree for gall stones; add guelder rose or wild yam to help relieve spasmodic pain.
- Precautions: Avoid pregnancy.

2. Citrus x limon—**LEMON**

Juice

- Actions: Used in traditional treatments with olive oil to break down and encourage excretion of gallstones; liver tonic and restorative.
- After fasting for the day, how to use: take 50 ml of olive oil and the juice of lemons in water at 6 p.m. Repeat three

times over the next hour. Bile sand is passed in stools over the following three days.

- Combinations: With Olive Oil.

Indigestion & Acidity

Usually due to eating too much, too quickly, missing meals, or anxiety. Antacids actually encourage further stomach acid secretion and can worsen the condition.

Key Symptoms

- Bloating and feelings of abdominal fullness.
- Heartburn or acid reflux.
- Stomach pain.

Remedies

1. Mentha x Piperita—**PEPPERMINT**

Aerial Parts

- Actions: Cooling carminative to ease flatulence and heartburn; stimulates bile flow; good for nervous tummies and nausea.
- How to use: 15 g of dried herb to 500 ml water in infusions; up to 2.5 ml tincture per dose.
- Combinations: Use as a simple; add American cranesbill to reduce acid secretions; add marshmallow root or licorice for inflammation.
- Precautions: May reduce milk flow; use with caution if breastfeeding.

2. Melissa officinalis—**LEMON BALM**

Aerial Parts

- Actions: Carminative and relaxing; sedative action so useful for nervous tummies.
- How to use: Standard infusion or tincture.
- Combinations: Add chamomile or fennel as anti-inflammatories or 10–20 drops of hop tincture as a bitter stimulant.

3. Foeniculum vulgare—**FENNEL**

Seeds

- Actions: Carminative and anti-inflammatory, effective for griping pains.
- How to use: Standard infusion or tincture useful as an after-dinner tisane.
- Combinations: Use as a simple; add American cranesbill to reduce acid secretions; add marshmallow root or licorice for inflammation.

Irritable Bowel Syndrome & Colitis

A convenient medical label for various digestive symptoms is often associated with anxiety, food intolerance, or infection.

Key Symptoms

- Alternating bouts of diarrhea and constipation.
- Characteristic "rabbit dropping" stools.

- Bloating and flatulence.
- Mucous in stools.

Remedies

1. Dioscorea villosa—**WILD YAM**

Rhizome

- Actions: Visceral relaxant and antispasmodic, anti-inflammatory, and bile stimulant.
- How to use: In decoctions (1 teaspoon to 500 m water) or combined with other tinctures.
- Combinations: Add meadowsweet to soothe gastric mucosa; chamomile or lemon balm if stress is an issue; or a few drops of fresh ginger tincture to help regulate bowel activity.
- Precautions: Avoid pregnancy or if trying to conceive.

2. Matricaria chamomilla—**GERMAN CHAMOMILE**

Flowers

- Actions: Sedative, anti-inflammatory, and carminative; good for nervous dyspepsia.
- How to use: Standard infusion or tincture.
- Combinations: Add a few drops of peppermint or fresh ginger tincture to relieve abdominal bloating and regulate bowel activity. Combine with lemon balm or passionflower if stress is a factor.

3. Iberis amaria—**BITTER CANDYTUFT**

Aerial Parts

- Actions: antispasmodic, relaxant, tonifies the digestive tract; carminative.
- How to use: Take up to 2 ml tincture per dose or an infusion made of 5 g herb to 500 ml water.
- Combinations: Add angelica root and milk thistle seeds as liver tonics; add chamomile or lemon balm if stress is an issue.
- Precautions: High doses may cause nausea.

Liver Disorders

In our polluted society, liver congestion is very common; it can manifest as pathological disorders but often involve feelings of anger and stagnation.

Key Symptoms

- The tendency for constipation.
- Abdominal bloating.
- Emotional lability.
- Menstrual disorders in women.
- Red, itching palms.
- Small petechiae on the abdomen.
- Sore, itching eyes.

Remedies

1. Bupleurum chinense—**CHAI HU**

Root

- Actions: Bitter liver tonic; stimulates bile flow, energy tonic, anti-inflammatory, and antibacterial.
- How to use: 10 g to 600 ml water for decoctions or up to 6 ml tincture daily.
- Combinations: Combine with bai Shao Yao, Chuanxiong, goldenseal, or dandelion in decoctions to improve liver function.

2. Silybum marianum—**MILK THISTLE**

Seeds

- Actions: Encourages liver cell renewal and repair; effective liver healer in degenerative conditions, including alcohol abuse.
- How to use: Standard infusion or up to 10 ml tincture daily.
- Combinations: Use as a simple or add vervain, gentian, dandelion root, or globe artichoke as additional liver tonics.

3. Picrorrhiza kurroa—**KATUKA ROOT**

- Actions: A traditional bitter Ayurvedic digestive remedy that protects the liver from various toxins and stimulates bile flow to help cleanse the gallbladder.
- How to use: Take 1 g per dose as a powder in capsules or mixed with ghee, or use half a teaspoon of crushed root for three doses of decoction.
- Combinations: Use other bitter digestive or liver stimulants such as turmeric, barberry, Gotu kola, and cardamom.
- Precautions: High doses may cause diarrhea, abdominal gripping, and flatulence; cases of allergic skin reaction have been reported.

Nausea & Vomiting

A symptom, rather than an identifiable disease, can be associated with various factors, including food poisoning, infections, fever, migraines, or pregnancy.

Note: Projectile or prolonged vomiting requires urgent professional medical help.

Remedies

1. Zingiber officinale—**GINGER**

Root

- Action: Very effective antiemetic useful for travel sickness as well as digestive upsets.
- How to use: Use standard tincture in drop doses on the tongue frequently while symptoms persist or chew crystallized ginger.
- Combinations: Use as a simple or combine with black horehound or chamomile tinctures Precautions: Use with care in early pregnancy.

2. Syzygium aromaticum—**CLOVES**

Flower Buds Or Essential Oil

- Actions: Stimulant and carminative also locally antiseptic.

- How to use: Standard infusion or use 1–2 drops of oil on a sugar lump internally; or sprinkle the powdered spice on food.
- Precautions: Do not exceed the stated dose of essential oil.

Flatulence & Abdominal Bloating

Often associated with minor digestive or liver problems, but can indicate serious illness.

Key Symptoms

- The wind may go up or down.
- Uncomfortable abdominal distention.

Remedies

1. Elettaria cardamomum—**CARDAMOM**

Seed Or Essential Oil

- Actions: Carminative and soothing for the digestive system; relieves abdominal cramps and stimulates appetite.
- How to use: Use the crushed seeds in infusions or tinctures; use 2–5 drops of essential oil in 5 ml of carrier oil for abdominal massage; use seeds in cooking.
- Combinations: Use soothing digestive remedies such as Gotu kola, fennel, chamomile, or lemon balm in infusions; add a pinch of galangal, ginger, or black pepper.

2. Cnicus benedictus—**HOLY THISTLE**

Flower Heads

- Actions: A bitter digestive stimulant that encourages stomach secretions and normalizes function.
- How to use: Use in infusions or tinctures.
- Combinations: Add lemon balm or chamomile with teas or centaury as an additional bitter; add carminatives such as a pinch of fennel seeds, black pepper, or cinnamon.
- Precautions: May cause vomiting in excessive doses.

Food Poisoning & Gastroenteritis

Gastric infection by viruses, bacteria, or protozoa may be due to pets, farm animals, or environmental hazards; food poisoning is a notifiable disease in some countries.

Key Symptoms

- Sudden onset with abdominal pain, nausea, and vomiting.
- Diarrhea, general malaise, and weakness.

Remedies

1. Matricaria chamomilla—**GERMAN CHAMOMILE**

Flowers

- Actions: Antimicrobial to combat infection, soothing and calming for the digestive system, reduces inflammation in the digestive tract.
- How to use: Use in infusions.

- Combinations: With astringents like agrimony or lady's mantle, soothing demulcents such as meadowsweet or marshmallow, and digestive tonics such as Gotu Kola. Add a pinch of ginger or cinnamon to combat nausea.

2. Alchemilla xanthoclora—LADY'S MANTLE

Leaves

- Actions: Astringent digestive tonic to reduce inflammation and discomfort.
- How to use: Use in infusions or tinctures.
- Combinations: With milk thistle seeds and marshmallow root to soothe the digestive tract and normalize function, eat garlic or take echinacea to combat infection.

Poor Appetite

Loss of appetite may be due to chronic illness, stress, or debility, all of which should also be treated.

Key Symptoms

- No interest in meals or eating.
- Weight loss and absence of menstruation in severe cases.

Note: Poor appetite may suggest eating disorders such as anorexia nervosa; seek immediate professional help if this is suspected.

Remedies

1. Trigonella foenum-graecum—**FENUGREEK**

Seeds

- Actions: Stimulating and tonifying for the whole digestive system; a traditional remedy for thin people hoping to put on weight.
- How to use: Take the seeds in infusions or use drops of the tincture on the tongue half an hour before meals.
- Combinations: Combine with milk thistle seeds or agrimony in infusions with a pinch of powdered ginger or galangal for

additional stimulation. Add chamomile, vervain, or wood betony if stress is a factor.

2. Jateorhiza calumba—**CALUMBA**

Root

- Actions: Bitter and stimulating for the digestive system; helps to relieve indigestion and normalize digestive function; stimulates the production of stomach acid.
- How to use: Use in macerations – half a cup, half an hour before meals, or take 20–40 drops of tincture in a little water before meals.
- Combinations: Combine with mugwort tincture in menstrual disorders or mix the maceration with agrimony, lemon balm, and chamomile infusions to soothe the digestive tract.
- Precautions: Avoid in pregnancy and gastric ulceration.

Halitosis/Bad Breath

Infections in the mouth, throat, lungs, or stomach can all contribute to bad breath; poor dental hygiene is often blamed.

Key Symptoms

- Stale or offensive breath.

Remedies

1. Levisticum officinale—**LOVAGE**

Seeds

- Actions: A tonic to normalize both digestive and respiratory function and improve the appetite; eases flatulence and combats bacteria; the seeds also contain aromatic oils.
- How to use: Chew a few seeds as required to freshen the breath and help normalize digestive function.
- Combinations: Mix with dill or fennel seeds if preferred; gargle with 5–10 drops of myrrh tincture in a glass of water

to help clear any mouth or gum infections; use appropriate remedies to treat any associated disorders contributing to the problem.

2. Iris versicolor—**BLUE FLAG**

Root

- Actions: Cleansing and stimulating for sluggish digestion, lymphatics, and glandular systems.
- How to use: Use powdered in capsules, 200 mg daily Combinations: Combine with powdered goldenseal, licorice, and echinacea or myrrh to combat underlying infections and congestion.

Hemorrhoids/Piles

Anal varicose veins are associated with poor muscle tone and often due to straining or constipation.

Key Symptoms

- Palpable piles at the anus.

- Bleeding on passing stool.

REMEDIES

1. Sophora japonica—**HUAI JIAO**

Fruit

- Actions: Cooling, anti-inflammatory, and hypotensive; clears liver heat, cools blood, and stops bleeding. Also helps constipation.
- How to use: Standard decoction or tincture; powdered in capsules (400 mg, three times a day).
- Combinations: Use as a simple or combine with liver tonics and digestive remedies such as dandelion root, barberry, dang gui, or zhi ke.
- Precautions: Avoid in pregnancy.

2. Ranunculus ficaria—**PILEWORT**

Root or Leaves

- Actions: Astringent to tonify blood vessels and stop bleeding.
- How to use: Apply ointment frequently.
- Combinations: Use as a simple but take supportive liver herbs or venous tonics
- such as king's clover. Take additional laxatives if need be to avoid constipation.
- Precautions: Do not take them internally.

ALLERGIC CONDITIONS

Allergies put the body under extra strain. The organism can cope with allergens when it is running well, but where there is added stress, infection, or exhaustion, the arrival of allergen tips the scale, resulting in an allergic reaction in the form of hay fever, gastric upsets, skin rashes, or other reactions.

When the immature gut has to deal with unfamiliar proteins, such as cow's milk, food allergies often begin in childhood. Inflammations, mucus, and irritation stimulate the immune system to repel the invader.

If the allergen is continued to be swallowed, the reaction becomes muted or masked over time. Although the allergen is still a burden on the body, there is no tell-tale rash or catarrh, only a general weakening of the immune system as it fights the allergen. This type of veiled allergy may present as ambiguous arthritic pains, irritable bowel syndrome, or chronic sinusitis, and diligent elimination diets may be required to pinpoint the source of the problem. Dairy items (usually cow's milk, but sometimes goat's or sheep's milk), as well as wheat gluten (found in wheat, barley, oats, and rye) and beef, are all known to trigger complications. Some fresh fruits, vegetables, and herbs contain salicylates, and daily use of aspirin-based medications seems to improve susceptibility to salicylates. Affected children can develop a rash after eating foods as diverse as strawberries, oranges, broccoli, mushrooms, tea, sweet corn, peanuts, and honey, making this a complicated allergy to diagnose.

It is best to remove the problematic foods once the digestive tract is soothed and healed as it comes to food intolerance. Gradually reintroduce them in a rotation schedule (no more than once per four days) to avoid toxic accumulation. Some allergens are difficult to prevent, such as house dust or pollen, and can be bothersome and permanent. Again, the herbal solution focuses on bolstering the respiratory and immune systems so that the allergen does not cause the typical reaction.

Hay Fever/Allergic Rhinitis

Hay fever is caused by grass or tree pollens which happens when these pollens are abundant. Allergies of house dust, cats, and other allergens exist year-round, with little seasonal variation.

Key Symptoms

- Copious nasal catarrh.
- Sore, irritated eyes.
- Sneezing.
- Severe cases can produce asthma-like symptoms.

Remedies

1. Euphrasia Officinalis—**EYEBRIGHT**

Aerial Parts

- Actions: Decreases nasal secretions and soothes mucous membranes and conjunctiva.
- How to use: Standard infusion, tincture, or two 200 mg capsules three times daily; also use 5 drops of tincture in an eye bath of water.
- Combinations: Combine with goldenseal powder in capsules; with elderflower in infusions or tinctures. Often prescribed with ma huang, which is a restricted herb in some geographies.

2. Glechoma hederacea—**GROUND IVY**

Aerial Parts

- Actions: Astringent and anti-catarrhal to dry secretions and inflammations.
- How to use: Standard infusion or tincture.

- Combinations: Combine with anti-catarrhals, such as marsh cudweed, in tinctures; take chamomile in infusions or use steam inhalants.

3. Plantago lanceolata—**RIBWORT PLANTAIN**

Leaves

- Actions: Good for allergic rhinitis, toning mucous membranes, and healing inflammations.
- How to use: Standard infusion or up to 4 ml of the tincture three times daily.
- Combinations: Add astringent anti-catarrhals such as marsh cudweed or ground ivy. Take chamomile in infusions or use steam inhalants.

Food Intolerance

Cow's milk, wheat, and beef are all common food allergens that can cause a wide variety of symptoms. Candidiasis, which is caused by a yeast overgrowth in the gut, may also be linked to food intolerance. Allergy to salicylates (aspirins, etc.) is becoming more widespread. Coeliac disease (gluten intolerance) may have serious health consequences.

Key Symptoms

- Digestive upsets – often diarrhea and flatulence.
- Stiffness and joint pain.
- Skin rashes and eczema.
- Respiratory problems, including asthma.
- Persistent urinary infections or vaginal thrush in candidiasis.
- Candidiasis can also be related to nervous disorders.

Remedies

1. Calendula officinalis—**POT MARIGOLD**

Flower Petals

- Actions: Antifungal and useful for excess yeasts in the gut in candidiasis.

- How to use: Use standard infusion or tincture well diluted in water.
- Combinations: Combine with elderflowers and agrimony or add antimicrobials such as echinacea in candidiasis or nervines if stress is an issue.

2. Hydrastis canadensis—**GOLDENSEAL**

Root

- Actions: Good liver stimulant and helps to ease gastric sensitivity; astringent and healing for the mucosa.
- How to use: Use in capsules – two 200 mg up to three times daily or in 2–4 ml tincture doses.
- Combinations: With powdered fenugreek or agrimony in capsules, with licorice in tinctures to soothe and heal mucous membranes.
- Precautions: Avoid in pregnancy and high blood pressure; do not exceed the stated dose.

3. Allium sativa—**GARLIC**

Cloves

- Actions: Antifungal, useful for excess yeasts in the gut and supports recovery of gut flora.
- How to use: Use 1 clove a day in cooking or take two 200 mg capsules.
- Combinations: Best as simple or with parsley to reduce the garlic odor.

4. Agrimonia eupatoria—**AGRIMONY**

Aerial Parts

- Actions: Soothes gut irritation and inflammation and heals damaged mucosa.
- How to use: Use standard infusion or up to 4 ml of tincture three times daily.
- Combinations: Add lemon balm and chamomile to reduce stress. Combine with soothing demulcents such as marshmallow root and take garlic or echinacea as antifungals.

Urtica/Hives

Blisters and rashes on the skin are caused by specific allergens, such as peanuts or chemical contact. Rashes are usually transient, but they can also be serious and long-lasting. It may be linked to a salicylate allergy.

Key Symptoms

- Irritant red swellings on the skin.

Note: Severe reactions and swelling can make it difficult to breathe or cause anaphylactic shock, which can be fatal; seek immediate medical attention.

1. Urtica dioica—**STINGING NETTLE**

Aerial Parts

- Actions: Taking nettles for nettle rash may seem a contradiction, but it can reduce itching and act as an antihistamine.

- How to use: Use infusions, tinctures or take two 200 mg capsules of powdered herb.
- Combinations: Use red clover, wood betony, and meadowsweet in infusions; add 20 drops of ma huang tincture dose to reduce the allergic reaction.
- Precautions: Ma huang is restricted in some geographies and may only be available on prescription.

2. Viola tricolor—**HEARTSEASE**

Aerial Parts

- Actions: Anti-inflammatory and soothing for any skin inflammation.
- How to use: Standard infusion or up to 15 ml of tincture daily, also as a wash or in ointments and creams.
- Combinations: Add 1–2 drops of thyme oil to 20 ml heartsease cream or add stinging nettle to infusions and tinctures.

3. Brassica oleracea—**CABBAGE**

Leaves

- Actions: Anti-inflammatory and healing; useful standby for emergencies.
- How to use: Apply a fresh leaf directly to the affected part or extract the juice and use it as a lotion.
- Combinations: Use as a simple. Fresh slices of onion can be similarly used.

Urinary Disorders

The kidneys and urinary system also represent an individual's overall wellbeing – something that chronic cystitis sufferers are well aware of since their symptoms worsen at periods of discomfort or exhaustion. Recurrent urinary infections, including recurrent colds, may signify a weakened immune system; tonic herbs and immune stimulant herbs are often required after the symptoms have subsided. A urinary antiseptic is usually used in herbal therapies since it includes volatile oils that tolerate ingestion, migrate through the bloodstream, and are excreted by the kidneys. To help relieve pain and restore damage to the mucosa, soothing demulcent herbs are applied to urinary tract treatments. Diuretics can also improve the flow to clean out the toxins and bacteria that have died.

In Chinese medicine, urinary inflammations are treated as heat and moist issues rather than bacterial infections. They are treated with soothing herbs like Huang qin, Zhi zie, ze Xie, mu tong, sheng di Huang, or rhubarb root (da Huang). Since the kidney and the urinary bladder are linked organs in traditional Chinese theory, a lack of kidney energy (qi) may contribute to bladder problems. Tonic herbs such as Huang qi, dang gui, ginseng, or bai zhu can be prescribed if you have excessive or nocturnal urination, incontinence, or the kind of dribbling after urination that we associate with classic prostate disease.

Urinary Tract Infections & Cystitis/Urethritis

Bladder inflammation (cystitis) in women and urethritis in men are the most common symptoms of urinary tract infections. Kidney involvement is possible in some cases, and it may be serious.

Key Symptoms

- Pain or burning sensation on passing water.
- Possible blood, mucus, or pus in the urine.
- Increased frequency of urination.
- Fever (more likely the higher up the urinary tract is the infection).
- Pain – may be located from groin to mid-back, depending on the site of infection.

NB: Both cases of kidney disease must be referred to a medical professional. If the source is venereal, cases must be referred to a specialist under UK legislation.

Remedies

1. Agathosma betulina—**BUCHU**

Leaves

- Actions: Diuretic and urinary antiseptic also have a warming and stimulant effect on the kidneys.

- How to use: 15 g of herb to 500 ml in infusion or up to 2 ml of tincture, or three 200 mg capsules three times daily.
- Combinations: Add couchgrass and yarrow to infusions or capsules. Add corn silk to soothe severe burning sensations.

2. Arctostaphylos uva-ursi—**BEARBERRY**

Leaves

- Actions: Produces potent antiseptic in the kidney tubules; effective with acid urine; how to use: 5 g of herb to 500 ml in infusion or up to 2 ml of the tincture three times daily.
- Combinations: Add couchgrass and yarrow to infusions; use horsetail juice or pellitory if there is damage to the mucosa.
- Precautions: High doses may cause nausea.

3. Apium graveolens—**CELERY**

Seed

- Actions: Urinary antiseptic and cleanses uric acid from the system.
- How to use: Standard infusion or up to 4 ml tincture three times daily.
- Combinations: Use horsetail, corn silk, or couchgrass to soothe inflamed mucosa.
- Precautions: Avoid in pregnancy; do not use seeds prepared for the garden trade.

4. Elymus repens—**COUCHGRASS**

Rhizome

- Actions: Contains mannitol, which is a diuretic, mucilages to soothe the mucosa, and is mildly antibiotic.
- How to use: Standard infusion or tincture.
- Combinations: Use buchu, bearberry, or juniper as more potent antiseptics.

Urinary Gravel

Deposits of insoluble content – either calcium salts or small uric acid crystals – develop in the bladder and may be linked to increases in urinary acidity or alkalinity.

Key Symptoms

- The sensation of "grittiness" on passing urine.
- Blood in urine in severe cases.
- Pain, which can be severe, between "loin and groin."

Remedies

1. Eupatorium purpureum—GRAVELROOT

Root

- Actions: Diuretic and soothing for the urinary mucosa useful for all irritations and inflammations.
- How to use: Use 20 g to 600 ml water in decoctions or up to 3 ml of the tincture three times daily.

- Combinations: Can be combined with parsley piert, corn silk, couchgrass, or pellitory-of-the-wall to soothe and encourage healing.

2. Parietaria diffusa—**PELLITORY-OF-THE-WALL**

Aerial Parts

- Actions: Diuretic and demulcent; useful for pain on urination; for kidney stones.
- How to use: Standard infusion or tincture; the fresh juice in 20 ml doses is particularly effective.
- Combinations: Add buchu or bearberry for infections; with couchgrass or corn silk to soothe and heal.

3. Juniperis communis—**JUNIPER**

Berries or Essential Oil

- Actions: Urinary antiseptic and diuretic; good for clearing acid wastes.

- How to use: Use 10 g of berries to 500 ml for infusions; up to 2 ml of tincture three times daily. Use the well-diluted oil as an abdominal massage.
- Combinations: Use parsley piert or hydrangea to help clear stones and add soothing remedies such as pellitory, cornsilk, or couchgrass.
- Precautions: Avoid in pregnancy and do not use continuously for more than six weeks without a break.

Kidney Stones

When insoluble calcium or oxalates develop in the kidney, they travel through the ureter and into the bladder, causing renal colic. Excess calcium intake can be related to stones.

Key Symptoms

- Agonizing "loin to groin" pain due to the passage of stones or gravel.

- Nausea, vomiting, blood in the urine.

Note: Always consult a professional practitioner.

Remedies

1. Aphanes arvensis—**PARSLEY PIERT**

Aerial Parts

- Actions: Also called parsley breakstone for its ability to break down stones in the kidney or bladder; diuretic, demulcent, and soothing for the urinary tract.
- How to use: Use in infusions or tinctures (up to 10 ml per dose).
- Combinations: Use hydrangea, ginger, and gravel root in tinctures, with cornsilk, pellitory of the wall, and khella (restricted in Australia) in infusions. Apply a hot compress of ginger to the lower abdomen if possible.

2. Amni visnaga—**KHELLA**

Seeds

- Actions: Relieves spasmodic pain by relaxing the muscles in the ureter, which helps ease the stone towards the bladder.
- How to use: Use in infusions or tinctures.
- Combinations: Use soothing demulcents such as cornsilk or marshmallow root; add shepherd's purse to help reduce any bleeding.
- Precautions: Restricted herb in Australia; prolonged or excessive use may cause nausea, headaches, and insomnia.

Nervous Disorders

A holistic approach to medicine prioritizes the needs of the body, mind, and spirit, particularly for conditions classified as "nerves." Physical manifestations of "nervous disorders" may include insomnia, palpitations, or headaches; emotional manifestations may include irritability, depression, and feelings of anger or guilt, whereas the lack of determination, emptiness, or a sense of purpose felt by so many people can typify the spiritual vacuum at the center of so many people's lives.

Herbs, like vervain, can be similarly holistic, working on the same three steps to promote well-being. It can be used as a liver tonic and a nervine relaxant. It is ideal for the perfectionist, slightly obsessive type who wants to do so many things at once and races each task to death like a dog worrying over a treat when taken as a Bach Flower Remedy. On a metaphysical basis, vervain can improve psychic perception and understanding: it was once used to lift consciousness in scurrying. Others believe it can heal gaps in the human aura (a layer of psychic energy that surrounds all living things).

Emotional imbalance is well accepted in Chinese and Ayurvedic medicine as a potential cause of the physical disease: the Chinese, for example, equate anxiety with the kidneys, so panic attacks may be a symptom of kidney imbalance or lead to kidney fatigue. Herbs may also enhance the chakras, which are thought to be the body's sacred centers in Eastern philosophy. Basil, for example, is thought to strengthen the root, second, and third chakras.

Herbal nerviness can thus work on many levels: they can be used in the same manner as traditional sedatives, hypnotics, or antidepressants, but they also have an emotional component that is familiar from the many flower and gem remedies now accessible. According to modern science, herbs can influence the mind and feelings in ways that we are just starting to learn. Aromatic compounds from essential oils, for example, pass through the olfactory system to access areas of the limbic region of the inner brain, which is responsible for thoughts and the processing and remembering of memories and perceptions.

Anxiety/Tension

Excessive life stresses can lead to a variety of health problems, not always obviously linked to tension.

Key Symptoms

- Inability to relax.
- Emotional lability – tendency to cry or be irritable for no obvious cause.
- Headaches.
- Sleeplessness.

Remedies

1. Stachys officinalis—**WOOD BETONY**

Aerial Parts

- Actions: Sedative and calming for the nervous system; good for nervous debility, fearfulness, and exhaustion.
- How to use: Standard infusion or tincture. It can be used powdered in capsules.
- Combinations: Good as a simple, or combine with chamomile, vervain, skullcap, or lavender to enhance tonic or sedative action.
- Precautions: Very large doses can be emetic.

2. Scutellaria lateriflora—**SKULLCAP**

Aerial Parts

- Actions: Relaxant and restorative for the central nervous system; good for nervous debility.

- How to use: Standard infusion or tincture or powdered in capsules.
- Combinations: Use as a simple or combine with wood betony, lavender, or lemon balm to increase calming, sedative action.

3. Tilia x Europaea—**LINDEN**

Flowers

- Actions: Reduces nervous tension and also helps prevent arteriosclerosis.
- How to use: Standard infusion or up to 10 ml of tincture daily.
- Combinations: Combines well with lemon balm and chamomile in infusions for an all-purpose relaxing tea.

4. Pulsatilla vulgaris—**PASQUE FLOWER**

Aerial Parts

- Actions: Nervine and anodyne with sedative action; useful for nervous tension and sexual problems.

- How to use: Up to 20 drops of tincture three times a day or use 5 g to 500 ml of water in infusions.
- Combinations: Add Jamaican dogwood or passionflower tincture for additional calming action.
- Precautions: Use only the dried plant as fresh is toxic.

5. Verbena officinalis—**VERVAIN**

Aerial Parts

- Actions: Relaxing nervine with a tonic effect on the liver.
- How to use: Use a standard infusion or tincture.
- Combinations: Use a simple combination with wood betony, linden, chamomile, or Gotu kola to enhance the sedative effect.
- Precautions: Avoid high doses in pregnancy.

Panic Attacks

It can be associated with excessive stress and also food intolerance. Severe cases may need psychiatric counseling.

Key Symptoms

- Palpitations.
- An intense feeling of fear.
- Feelings of impending doom.

Remedies

1. Rosa x Damascena—**DAMASK ROSE**

Essential Oil

- Actions: Very soothing for the nerves, antidepressant and antiemetic; gentle sedative.
- How to use: Add 5–10 drops of rose oil to 10 ml of carrier oil and use to massage temples or throat. Add 2–5 drops of essential oil to baths and use rosewater in lotions or cooking.
- Combinations: Can combine with a few drops of sandalwood or lavender oils to enhance the calming effect.

- Precautions: Do not take oils internally without professional advice. Rose oil is extremely expensive, and synthetic substitutes are commonplace; buy only good quality genuine rose oil.

2. Citrus aurantium—**NEROLI**

Essential Oil

- Actions: Sedative and antidepressant, traditionally used for hysteria, panic, and fearfulness. Eases palpitations and cardiac spasm.
- How to use: Add 5–10 drops of rose oil to 10 ml of carrier oil and use to massage temples or throat. Add 5–10 drops of essential oil to baths and use orange flower water in lotions or cooking.
- Combinations: Combine with 10 drops of lavender or benzoin oils to enhance calming action.
- Precautions: Do not take oils internally without professional advice.

3. Piscidia erythrina—**JAMAICAN DOGWOOD**

Bark

- Actions: Sedative and anodyne useful for severe nervous tension, insomnia, or nervous migraine.
- How to use: Use up to 5 ml tincture daily or in decoction with other herbs (use 5g of Jamaican dogwood and up to 15 g of others in 600 ml water).
- Combinations: Add pasque flower, valerian, or hop tinctures to give a combined total of up to 5 ml per dose for additional sedative action.
- Precautions: Do not exceed stated doses.

4. Hyssopus officinalis—**HYSSOP**

Aerial Parts or Essential Oil

- Actions: Antispasmodic and mildly analgesic, traditionally used for hysteria and some forms of epilepsy; it is also gentle enough for upsets in children.
- How to use: Take an infusion or tincture; use 2–3 drops of essential oil in almond oil to massage temples and neck.

- Combinations: Add skullcap, passionflower, or wood betony to infusions to enhance the sedating effect if desired.
- Precautions: Do not take oils internally without professional advice.

Depression

Debility of the nervous system is traditionally associated with a surfeit of the "melancholic" humor in Galenical medicine.

Key symptoms

- Poor digestive function with constipation.
- Misery, "feeling down."
- Inability to concentrate.
- Lack of interest in the present.
- Withdrawn, silent demeanor.

Remedies

1. Ocimum basilicum—**BASIL**

Leaves and Essential Oil

- Action: Antidepressant and spiritually uplifting, especially effective for the lower chakras – useful to encourage earthing and groundedness.
- How to use: Eat fresh leaves; use 5 drops of the oil in bathwater, or add to massage oils; take up to 3 ml of tincture per dose.
- Combinations: Combine leaves with lemon balm or rose petals in infusion; add a few drops of geranium or rose oils to massage mix to increase uplifting effects.
- Precautions: Do not take oils internally without professional advice; do not use the oil in pregnancy.

2. Avena sativa—**OATS**

Straw and Seeds

- Actions: Antidepressant and restorative nerve tonic.
- How to use: Use 2–3 ml wild oat fluid extract or standard decoction; eat oatmeal as porridge.
- Combinations: Combines well with vervain tincture or add 10 drops of lemon balm or St. John's wort tinctures per dose to enhance antidepressant action.

3. Borago officinalis—**BORAGE**

Leaves

- Actions: Restorative for the adrenal cortex, eases depression.
- How to use: Use 10 ml of juice three times daily.
- Combinations: Use as a simple.
- Precautions: Restricted herb in some geographies.

4. Turnera diffusa—**DAMIANA**

Aerial Parts

- Actions: Stimulating nervine (especially good for the male hormonal system); antidepressant.

- How to use: Use up to 2.5 ml of the tincture—three times daily or 20 g to 500 ml water for infusions.
- Combinations: Combine with oat tincture or fluid extract for general depression; add St. John's wort or wood betony tincture if anxiety is a problem to give a total combined dose of 5 ml.

Insomnia

It can be associated with over-excitement, anxiety, and worries, or some physical cause (such as pain) that needs treating. In Chinese, medicine can signify excessive "heart fire."

Key Symptoms

- Inability to fall asleep.
- Frequent wakefulness during the night.
- Restlessness, vivid dreamy sleep.

Remedies

1. Passiflora incarnates—**PASSION FLOWER**

Leaves

- Actions: Sedative, hypnotic and anodyne – calms the nervous system and promotes sleep.
- How to use: Take 5 ml of tincture 30 minutes before retiring at night or drink an infusion with 2 teaspoons dried leaves per cup.
- Combinations: Add lavender and chamomile to infusions if desired.
- Precautions: Avoid high doses in pregnancy.

2. Lactuca virosa—**WILD LETTUCE**

Leaves

- Actions: Sedative – the latex was once known as "poor man's opium" – the fresh herb is especially potent when it goes to seed (garden lettuce can have a similar but milder effect).

- How to use: Drink a cup of a standard infusion or up to 5 ml of tincture 30 minutes before retiring at night
- Combinations: Can be combined with additional calming herbs such as tinctures of passionflower, valerian, or cowslip petals to give a total of 5 ml of the combined tinctures per dose.
- Precautions: Large doses may cause confusion and stupor; may cause sudden sleepiness soon after ingestion, so avoid driving or using machinery.

3. Humulus lupulus—**HOPS**

Strobiles

- Action: Sedative, hypnotic and anodyne – calms excess excitability.
- How to use: Use up to 5 ml of tincture daily, or 10 g of the dried herb with 500 ml water for infusions.

- Combinations: Can be combined with additional calming herbs such as valerian or passionflower tinctures up to a maximum of 5 ml of the combined tinctures per dose.
- Precautions: Hops rapidly oxidize, and actions vary depending on the age of the herb.

4. Eschscholzia californica—**CALIFORNIA POPPY**

Aerial Parts

- Actions: Gentle and non-addictive hypnotic, tranquilizer and anodyne. Safe for children.
- How to use: Standard dose of infusion or tincture is taken before retiring at night.
- Combinations: Use as a simple combination with passionflower or lavender; add cowslip petals if over-excitability is a problem.

Inability to Relax

Herbs have long been used to induce relaxation and, in traditional societies, trance-like states with altered levels of awareness: tobacco and cannabis have still been used this way in the West.

Key Symptoms

- Restlessness, cannot sit still.
- Irritability, poor attention span.
- Constant chatter.

Remedies

1. Lavandula spp.—**LAVENDER**

Flowers & Essential Oil

- Actions: Sedative and analgesic with antispasmodic action.
- How to use: Take a standard infusion or up to 4 ml of tincture per dose. Massage diluted oil into temples.

- Combinations: Use as a simple or combine with wood betony, linden flowers, or vervain in infusions to ease tensions and stress.
- Precautions: Do not take lavender oil internally without professional guidance.

2. Chamaemelum nobile—**ROMAN CHAMOMILE**

Flowers & Essential Oil

- Actions: Sedative, carminative and antispasmodic. Good for excitement and nervous tummies.
- How to use: Add 2–3 drops of essential oil or 500 ml of infusion to baths; drink chamomile tea regularly.
- Combinations: Use as a simple or add lemon balm, skullcap, or Gotu kola to tinctures to relax and restore; combine with 2–3 drops of lavender oil in baths as an additional sedative.
- Precautions: Do not take essential oils internally without professional guidance.

3. Centella asiatica—**GOTU KOLA**

Aerial Parts

- Actions: Relaxing and restorative for the nervous system; good for neurotic disturbances.
- How to use: Take a standard infusion or tincture.
- Combinations: Use as a simple or mix with a little lavender or chamomile flowers in infusions to enhance calming action.
- Precautions: Best taken for short periods (4–6 weeks), then give a two-week break.

Emotional Upsets

Temper tantrums, mood swings, irritability, and grief – life's mental ups and downs affect people of all ages. Extracts (such as Bach Flower Remedies or Bush Essences) may also be beneficial.

Key Symptoms

- Irrational tears or anger with no apparent cause.

Remedies

1. Melissa officinalis—**LEMON BALM**

Leaves

- Actions: Antidepressant and restorative for the nervous system.
- How to use: Drink an infusion of fresh herbs as required or take up to 5 ml of tincture daily (it is more effective in low doses).
- Combinations: Use as a simple or combined with wood betony, skullcap, or vervain tinctures for sedative and restorative action.

2. Valeriana officinalis—**VALERIAN**

Root

- Actions: Very potent tranquilizer, antispasmodic and mild anodyne.

- How to use: Take a maceration or tincture, also available in 200 mg capsules or tablets.
- Combinations: Use as a simple or add a small number of hops if there is excitability—support with a massage using rose or lavender oils.
- Precautions: Can lead to over-excitedness in some individuals; try a small dose first to check for a reaction.

3. Artemisia vulgaris—**MUGWORT**

Aerial Parts

- Actions: Gentle nervine; useful for menopausal tensions and for mild depressions and stress.
- How to use: Take up to 2 ml (40 drops) of tincture three times a day or drink a weak infusion.
- Combinations: Combine with wood betony, skullcap, or vervain for menopausal tension with emotional stress; combine tinctures up to a total of 5 ml per dose.
- Precautions: Avoid in pregnancy and when breastfeeding.

Coping With Stress

Stress is a natural aspect of life that helps us stay alert and active; it causes the release of adrenaline, the "fight or flight" hormone; inability to react physically results in a "negative stress response" characterized by excessive physical tension.

Key Symptoms

- Dry mouth, easy tears, palpitations, or panic attacks.
- Constant tiredness, difficulty sleeping or concentrating,
- Inability to relax, headaches, muscular aches and pains, stomach upsets.

Remedies

1. Eleutherococcus senticosus—**SIBERIAN GINSENG**

Root

- Actions: Helps the body to cope more efficiently with stress and improves stamina; useful as a preventative before exams, a busy time at work, or long-haul air travel to combat jet lag.

- How to use: Take up to 600 mg a day for 10–14 days before the stresses are peaked. This can be useful stress preventative before exams.
- Combinations: Use as a simple of combine with reishi mushroom in capsules.

2. Matricaria chamomilla—**GERMAN CHAMOMILE**

Flowers

- Actions: Calming and mildly sedative to encourage relaxation and act as a tonic for the digestive system stress-related upsets.
- How to use: Use in infusions.
- Combinations: Combine with lemon balm or wood betony in infusions; add a few jasmine flowers to the mix if available.

Exhaustion & Tiredness

Often dismissed as a symptom but may be related to destructive emotions, overwork, or chronic illness.

Key Symptoms

- Difficulty getting out of bed each morning.
- Lacking the energy to complete tasks.
- Difficulty concentrating.

Important: Constant or excessive tiredness may be a sign of undiagnosed illness; seek professional help if symptoms have no apparent cause.

Remedies

1. Panax Ginseng—**KOREAN GINSENG**

Root

- Actions: Energy tonic, traditionally used in China for older people and ideal to help the body adjust to changing seasons.
- How to use: Best taken in periods of up to four weeks, 600 mg in capsules or tablets, or up to 10 ml of tincture daily.
- Combinations: Use as a simple or combine with huang qi, ginkgo, or ashwagandha and a little ginger or galangal.
- Precautions: Avoid long-term or excessive use in pregnancy; may add to macho aggression in young, very young men.

2. Salvia officinalis Purpurescens Group or Salvia officinalis—**PURPLE or GREEN SAGE**

Aerial Parts

- Actions: Restorative, hormonal, and antioxidant; stimulates the nervous and digestive systems.
- How to use: Take in infusion, tinctures, or powdered in capsules (up to 1 g daily).

- Combinations: Use rosemary, Gotu kola, wood betony, hibiscus, or thyme in infusions.
- Precautions: Avoid high doses in pregnancy and completely in epilepsy.

Chronic Fatigue Syndrome

The issue has been attributed to viral infection, immune deficiency, and psychiatric disturbances and is known as a post-viral syndrome or myalgic encephalomyelitis (ME).

Key Symptoms

- Muscle fatigue and weakness after even minor exercise.
- Headaches, muscular pains, breathing problems.
- Weariness and difficulty concentrating.

Remedies

1. Astragalus membranaceous—**HUANG QI**

Root

- Actions: Stimulating for both the immune system and energy levels; traditionally used in China for younger people affected by ME.
- How to use: Use tinctures, decoction, or powdered in capsules (up to 600 mg daily).
- Combinations: With ginseng and echinacea; support with evening primrose oil, zinc, and vitamin C supplements, and Gotu Kola, milk thistle, and cardamom in infusions.

2. Withania somnifera—**ASHWAGANDHA**

Root

- Actions: A nutritive and rejuvenating tonic to act on both physical and mental energies.
- How to use: In tinctures, decoctions, or 250 mg to 1 g of powder per dose in capsules or with a little water; take up to 5 g daily in warm milk sweetened with a little sugar.
- Combinations: Add a long little pepper to enhance action; combine with ginseng and licorice in decoctions. Support with liver stimulants and 25 ml daily of cleavers juice to

cleanse the lymphatic system. Eat plenty of shiitake mushrooms to help the immune system.

3. Echinacea spp.—**Echinacea**

Root or Leaves

- Actions: Antiviral and antifungal to combat associated infection and possible candidiasis.
- How to use: In tinctures or capsules (two 200 mg, three times daily); in decoction or infusion depending on part used.
- Combinations: Combine with cleavers, milk thistle, and galangal tinctures; use in infusions with Gotu kola and decoctions with huang qi or ginseng. Support with evening primrose, zinc, and vitamin C supplements as before.
- Precautions: High doses may rarely cause dizziness and nausea.

Seasonal Affective Disorder (Sad)

Depression and emotional problems associated with short daylight hours and dark winter days. Often helped by special artificial daylight lighting systems.

Key Symptoms

- Clear seasonal association with depression.
- Insomnia, weariness, occasional sugar cravings.

Remedies

1. Hypericum perforatum—**ST. JOHN'S WORT**

Aerial Parts

- Actions: Proven anti-depressive is increasingly used as an alternative to orthodox drugs.
- How to use: In tinctures, teas, or capsules.
- Combinations: Use with wood betony, basil, or lemon balm infusions or tinctures.

- Precautions: Reports suggest long-term or excessive use may be associated with cataracts.

2. Rosmarinus officinalis—**ROSEMARY**

Aerial Parts Or Essential Oil

- Actions: Stimulating for the nervous system, antioxidant, and tonifying for digestion.
- How to use: Take the fresh or dried leaves in infusions or tinctures; use 5–10 drops of oil in bathwater.
- Combinations: Mix with basil, sage, and thyme for a stimulating and uplifting tea; add 2–3 drops of rose geranium oil to baths.

Shock

Emotional shock is associated with sudden fears; physical shock may follow traumatic accidents.

Key Symptoms

- Cold sweat, palpitations, breathlessness, shivering, confusion.

Remedies

1. Capsicum frutescens—**CAYENNE**

Fruit

- Actions: Stimulates blood circulation and tissues throughout the body; warming, restorative and normalizing.
- How to use: Take up to 5 drops of tincture in a little water or directly to the tongue.
- Combinations: Use the drops of tincture in a cup of sage or chamomile infusion. Drink plenty of fluids.

2. Alpinia spp.—**GALANGAL**

Root

- Actions: Warming and stimulating; especially effective for calming palpitations, irregular heartbeat, and feelings of panic.
- How to use: Take up to 5 drops of tincture directly to the tongue; use in a decoction Combinations: Use the drops of tincture in a cup of skullcap infusion; drink plenty of fluids.

Use of Marijuana in Herbalism

Even though every state has regulations prohibiting the use of medical marijuana, more than two-thirds of states and the District of Columbia have done so, and more are proposing legislation to do so. Even though many patients use marijuana, it is only licensed by the FDA to treat two unusual and serious cases of epilepsy, Dravet syndrome, and Lennox-Gastaut syndrome.

Why has not there been further testing done? One explanation is that marijuana is classified as a Schedule I substance by the US Drug Enforcement Administration (DEA), along with opium, LSD, and ecstasy, meaning it is very likely to be abused and has little medicinal use. According to Marcel Bonn-Miller, Ph.D., a drug misuse expert at the University of Pennsylvania Perelman School of Medicine, scholars require a special certification to study it.

That is unlikely to improve shortly. The Law Enforcement Administration proposed reclassifying marijuana as a Schedule II drug, similar to Ritalin or oxycodone, but instead opted to retain it as a

Schedule I drug. However, the department agreed to fund more marijuana testing to make the procedure simpler for researchers. "Research is critically needed because we have to be able to advise patients and doctors on the safe and effective use of cannabis," Bonn-Miller says.

He had some insight into the benefits of medical marijuana as well as possible side effects.

What Is Medical Marijuana?

Medical marijuana is used to cure illnesses or disorders by using the marijuana plant or its chemicals. It is almost the same as recreational marijuana, although it is used for medicinal reasons.

Cannabinoids are a group of chemicals found in marijuana plants that number in the hundreds. Each has a distinct effect on the human body. The key chemicals used in medicine are delta-9-tetrahydrocannabinol (THC) and cannabidiol (CBD). When people smoke marijuana or eat foods containing THC, they experience a "high."

What Is Medical Marijuana Used For?

Legal marijuana is being researched to see how it can assist with a variety of ailments:

- Alzheimer's disease
- Appetite loss
- Cancer
- Crohn's disease
- Diseases affecting the immune system like HIV/AIDS or Multiple Sclerosis (MS)
- Eating disorders such as anorexia
- Epilepsy
- Glaucoma
- Mental health conditions like schizophrenia and posttraumatic stress disorder (PTSD)
- Multiple sclerosis
- Muscle spasms
- Nausea

- Pain
- Seizures
- Wasting syndrome (cachexia)

With a few exceptions, Bonn-Miller notes, it has not yet been shown to help all of these diseases. "The greatest amount of evidence for the therapeutic effects of cannabis relate to its ability to reduce chronic pain, nausea and vomiting due to chemotherapy, and spasticity [tight or stiff muscles] from MS," Bonn-Miller claims.

How Does It Help?

Cannabinoids, the active ingredients of medical marijuana, are related to hormones that regulate appetite, memory, breathing, and pain in the body.

Cannabinoids, according to limited evidence, may:

- Reduce the stress levels.
- Relieve discomfort and reduce inflammation

- Control cancer chemotherapy-induced nausea and vomiting.
- Cancer cells are killed, and tumor development is slowed.
- People with MS should relax their tense muscles.
- In cancer and AIDS, patients stimulate appetite and help them gain weight.

Can Medical Marijuana Help With Seizure Disorders?

When parents said that a special form of medical marijuana helped control epilepsy in their children a few years ago, it drew a lot of attention. Epidiolex, a CBD-based therapy, was recently approved by the FDA to treat people with serious or difficult-to-treat epilepsy. Any people had a significant reduction in epilepsy after taking this prescription, according to reports.

Has The FDA Approved Medical Marijuana?

Epidiolex, a cannabinoid, was used in 2018 to treat seizures associated with Lennox-Gastaut syndrome and Dravet syndrome, two uncommon and extreme cases of epilepsy. Furthermore, the FDA has approved the use of dronabinol (Marinol, Syndros) and nabilone (Cesamet) to relieve nausea and vomiting caused by chemotherapy. Epidiolex, a cannabinoid, was used in 2018 to treat seizures associated with Lennox-Gastaut syndrome and Dravet syndrome, two uncommon and extreme cases of epilepsy.

How Do You Take It?

To take medical marijuana, you can:

- Smoke it
- Inhale it through a device called a vaporizer that turns it into a mist

- Eat it -- for example, in a brownie or lollipop
- Apply it to your skin in a lotion, spray, oil, or cream
- Place a few drops of a liquid under your tongue

It is all up to you how you handle it. Each procedure affects the body in a particular way. "If you smoke or vaporize cannabis, you feel the effects very quickly," Bonn-Miller says. "It takes much longer if you eat it. The results of edible items can take anywhere from 1 to 2 hours to manifest."

What Are The Side Effects Of Medical Marijuana?

Side effects that have been reported include:

- Bloodshot eyes
- Depression
- Dizziness
- Fast heartbeat
- Hallucinations

- Low blood pressure

The medication can impair judgment and coordination, potentially resulting in accidents and injuries. Marijuana usage during adolescence, when the brain is still evolving, can affect IQ and mental performance. There have been fears that smoking marijuana could damage the lungs because it contains some of the same chemicals as tobacco. While the effects of inhaled marijuana on lung health are unknown, there is some evidence that it may raise the risk of bronchitis and other lung issues.

Marijuana, according to the National Institute on Opioid Abuse, can be addictive and is a "gateway drug" for other drugs. "The higher the level of THC and the more often you use, the more likely you are to become dependent," Bonn-Miller says. "If you need to rest, you find it impossible to do so. When you are not used, you experience cravings. To have the same impact, you will need more and more of it." See more about marijuana's long-term consequences.

Another problem is that medical marijuana is not controlled by the FDA in the same way that prescription drugs are. While states have the authority to oversee and control transactions, they cannot also do so. As a result, the potency and additives of medical marijuana can vary greatly depending on where you purchase it. "Last year, we conducted a report in which we bought labeled edible items in California and Washington, such as brownies and lollipops. Then we took them to the laboratory, "According to Bonn-Miller. "Few of the items contained anything close to what they said. That is a problem."

Which States Allow Medical Marijuana?

Medical marijuana is legal in 33 states and the District of Columbia:

- Alaska
- Arizona
- Arkansas
- California
- Colorado
- Connecticut
- Delaware
- District of Columbia

- Florida
- Hawaii
- Illinois
- Louisiana
- Maine
- Maryland
- Massachusetts
- Michigan
- Minnesota
- Missouri
- Montana
- Nevada
- New Hampshire
- New Jersey
- New Mexico
- New York
- North Dakota
- Ohio
- Oklahoma

- Oregon
- Pennsylvania
- Rhode Island
- Utah
- Vermont
- Washington
- West Virginia

States allowing legal recreational use include Alaska, California, Colorado, Illinois, Maine, Massachusetts, Michigan, Nevada, Oregon, Vermont, and the Washington States that allow restricted use only include: Alabama, Georgia, Idaho, Iowa, Kentucky, Mississippi, Missouri, North Carolina, South Carolina, Tennessee, Texas, Virginia, Wisconsin, and Wyoming.

How Do You Get Medical Marijuana?

In states where medical marijuana is legal, you would require a written prescription from a registered doctor to obtain it. (Not all doctors are comfortable recommending medical marijuana to their patients.) You must have a medical condition that allows you to use medical marijuana. - state has its own set of eligibility requirements. Your state may ask you to obtain a medical marijuana identification card. You can get medical marijuana from a pharmacy if you have your card.

When and Why You Should Consult an Herbalist

Although many people use herbs as natural and reliable home remedies for mild aches and pains, chronic or more severe issues, need clinical assistance. Finding a doctor with whom you can empathize and trust is almost as vital as taking the right herbs when it comes to therapy. Some herbalists use a more traditional approach, prescribing remedies to alleviate symptoms, while others rely on natural approaches and recommend significant lifestyle adjustments. Some will only use Western spices, while others will combine Chinese and Ayurvedic medicines. Some will discuss clinical disorders only, while others may mention qi stagnation, allergies, or emotional tension.

If at all practicable, select your doctor based on personal recommendations from like-minded peers to maintain a positive friendship with someone who cares and can communicate with you. Alternatively, request a registry of representatives from the national regulatory authority and consult with potential physicians before scheduling an appointment. Inquire into their expertise handling ailments close to yours and their general clinical method. Infections, aches, pains, menstrual complications, elevated blood pressure, urinary dysfunction, or intestinal issues are typical ailments treated, as are chronic diseases like rheumatoid arthritis, ME, or emphysema, for which herbalism is often used. As a "last resort."

Who Are The Herbalists?

Around the globe, national practices and laws differ. The National Institute of Medical Herbalists, established in 1864 in the United Kingdom, is the world's oldest independent organization of medical herbalists. Before being admitted into membership, students must undergo several years of study, which today entails a degree course in herbal medicine from an approved university and 500 hours of supervised clinical training. Members' names are preceded by the letters MNIMH or FNIMH, which gives patients some assurance that they are seeing a well-qualified practitioner. In 1989, well-known herbalist Michael Tierra founded the American Herbalists Guild in the United

States. Like those of the NIMH, membership requirements are stringent, requiring four years of graduate study and 400 hours of clinical experience. RH(AHG) (registered herbalist AHG)" is a common abbreviation used by practitioners. Finding out about the essence of your preferred practitioner's training can be simple, thanks to the AHG website, which lists the various colleges in the United States that deliver herb courses and their graduates' credentials. The education of practitioners can be easy.

In France, herbal practitioners, or phytothérapeutes, are almost all trained doctors who have studied plant medicine at a post-graduate level; in Germany, alternative practitioners are known as "heilpraktiker" and have the same status as orthodox GPs; and in many Eastern European medical schools, "materia medica," or the study of herbal remedies, is taught. In Australia, qualified herbalists join the National Herbalists Association as full members and use the initials NHAA after their names. The Commonwealth Government has designated them as Health Care Professionals.

Traditional herbal medicine is taught in dedicated colleges. It is accessible to patients as an alternative to Western medicine at special hospitals in China, whereas herbal treatments are available on Japan's equivalent to the National Health Service. Other countries, including some US states, make it illegal to administer herbal medicines or set up shop as a herbal practitioner, though self-medication with herbs is legal. In some, anybody, well-trained or not, can set up shop as a medical herbalist and prescribe all sorts of ineffective "treatments."

What Does An Herbalist Do?

An herbalist can use patient listening and probing questions and time-honored medical procedures such as sensing breaths, checking at tongues, measuring urine and blood pressure, and clinical tests based on palpation auscultation and percussion to reveal any possible signs during a visit. A first consultation will typically last at least an hour, with additional consultations lasting about 20 minutes. As well as reviewing the current illness, the herbalist will ask about medical history – previous health problems that may be contributing to the current imbalance, family tendencies and allergies, diet, lifestyle, stresses, and worries. It is, therefore, a good idea to double-check all existing orthodox medications. Herbalists do not advocate discontinuing life-saving medications, but any incompatibility of herbal therapies must be considered while administering plant medicines. Similarly, many people resort to herbs because they want to wean themselves off of their medications for some purpose. A health plan for replacing them with gentler herbal therapies must be formulated – ideally with the patient's GP's encouragement and cooperation.

Many herbalists also dispense their own medicines, so the patient can leave with a selection of suitable tinctures, ointments, or capsules – or even a bag of dried herbs to brew at home – after the appointment. Whatever the treatment, it would have been carefully chosen to benefit the patient's welfare. Regardless of the treatment, it would have been hand-picked to address the specific health concerns of the customer, rather than being a generic range of ready-made drugs. Herbalists want to see patients shortly after the first appointment to report for results – maybe two to three weeks afterward – with follow-up visits of four to six weeks for three months or longer in chronic conditions. To indicate improvements in the disorder, herbal medicine is likely to be tweaked slightly after each consultation. Healing is a two-way operation, and the patient must take responsibility for their own recovery and actively engage in the cure, just as all patients are different.

References

Kennedy, A. (2017). *Herbal Medicine Natural Remedies: 150 Herbal Remedies to Heal Common Ailments*. Althea Press.

Shimer, P. (2004). *Healing Secrets of the Native Americans: Herbs, Remedies, and Practices That Restore the Body, Refresh the Mind, and Rebuild the Spirit*. Black Dog & Leventhal.

Aniys, A. (2016). *Alkaline Herbal Medicine: Reverse Disease and Heal the Electric Body*. CreateSpace Independent Publishing Platform.

Chevallier, A. (2016). *Encyclopedia of Herbal Medicine: 550 Herbs and Remedies for Common Ailments* (3rd edition). DK.

Ody, P. (2017). *The Complete Medicinal Herbal: A Practical Guide to the Healing Properties of Herbs* (Reprint ed.). Skyhorse.

Farr, S. (2016). *Healing Herbal Teas: Learn to Blend 101 Specially Formulated Teas for Stress Management, Common Ailments, Seasonal Health, and Immune Support*. Storey Publishing, LLC.

Sams, T. (2015). *Healing Herbs: A Beginner's Guide to Identifying, Foraging, and Using Medicinal Plants / More than 100 Remedies from 20 of the Most Healing Plants* (1st ed.). Fair Winds Press.

Rn, R. K. (2014). *Herbal Antibiotics: Beginners Guide to Using Herbal Medicine to Prevent, Treat and Heal Illness with Natural Antibiotics and Antivirals.* CreateSpace Independent Publishing Platform.

Jones, M. (2017). *Herbal Antibiotics: What BIG Pharma Doesn't Want You to Know - How to Pick and Use the 45 Most Powerful Herbal Antibiotics for Overcoming Any Ailment.* Createspace Independent Publishing Platform.

Swift, K., & Midura, R. (2018). *Herbal Medicine for Beginners: Your Guide to Healing Common Ailments with 35 Medicinal Herbs* (1st ed.). Althea Press.

Dugliss-Wesselman, S., & Gregg, S. (2018). *Herbal Remedies Made Simple: A Beginner's Guide to Using Plants, Herbs, and Flowers for Health and Well-Being.* Fair Winds Press.

Hoffmann, D. (2003). *Medical Herbalism: The Science Principles and Practices Of Herbal Medicine* (Illustrated ed.). Healing Arts Press.

Jones, M. (2015). *The Complete Guide to Creating Oils, Soaps, Creams, and Herbal Gels for Your Mind and Body 101 Natural Body Care Recipes Revised 2nd Edition (Back to Basics)* (2nd Revised ed.). Atlantic Publishing Group Inc.

Cnc, P. B. A. (2010). *Prescription for Nutritional Healing, Fifth Edition: A Practical A-to-Z Reference to Drug-Free Remedies Using Vitamins, Minerals, Herbs & Food . . . A-To-Z Reference to Drug-Free Remedies)* (5th Revised, Updated ed.). Avery.

Shealy, N. C. (2012). *The Healing Remedies Sourcebook: Over 1000 Natural Remedies to Prevent and Cure Common Ailments* (1st ed.). Da Capo Lifelong Books.

Bremness, L. (1994). *The Complete Book of Herbs: A Practical Guide to Growing and Using Herbs*. Studio.

Phillips, N., Phillips, M., & Gladstar, R. (2005). *The Herbalist's Way: The Art and Practice of Healing with Plant Medicines* (Revised ed.). Chelsea Green Publishing.

Made in United States
Troutdale, OR
11/03/2026

56847398R00159